BEYOND FASTING

Strategies for Extraordinary Health and Longevity

Dr. Daniel Pompa

Published by Revelation Health, LLC

BEYOND FASTING

Strategies for Extraordinary Health and Longevity Printed in the United States of America.

ISBN 978-1-7337131-0-8

Dedicated to Merily, my wife, the love of my life,
and the most extraordinary person I know.

TABLE OF CONTENTS

FOREWORD BY BEN GREENFIELD

Dr. Pompa is not only a colleague with a shared interest in helping people to heal at the cellular level, but he is also a close friend of mine. My dear friend, Dr. Isaac Jones, introduced me to Dr. Pompa.

I was in the backcountry of Utah taking part in a bow hunting and obstacle course racing competition. Dr. Pompa and his wife, Merily, were kind enough to allow my sore, bedraggled, and bloodied body into their home to recover after the event. That recovery was complete with organic wine, grass- fed steak, detoxification, and all manner of bio-hacking geekery. I realized right then I'd met a true kindred spirit and a man who shares my passion for innovative techniques geared towards total optimization of the mind, body, and spirit.

He has an interesting story too. After years of struggling with chronic illness, Dr. Pompa rebuilt his health from the ground up. Since then, he has worked directly with sick clients from all over the world to help them do the same. Over the past decade, he has become a well-recognized expert on topics like fasting, diet variation, and cellular detoxification. He has collaborated with some of the world's greatest health professionals, scientists, and enthusiasts. Together through studying the scientific literature, clinical observation, and self-experimentation, he and his colleagues have put together what I consider to be some very innovative protocols for maximizing health and longevity.

Dr. Pompa is mainly known for his *True Cellular Detox* (TCD) program, which is a safe and comprehensive approach to detoxification. He also leads a nationwide network of functional medicine doctors called Health Centers of the Future (HCF), through which these protocols are implementing into hundreds of private practices across the U.S. Thousands of people around the world have been able to benefit from his body of work through his website, social media, podcasts, and doctors.

Today, there are millions of people around the world suffering from the symptoms of premature aging and chronic degenerative diseases. We see epidemics of metabolic and inflammatory-based illnesses, such as cancers, auto-immune conditions, Alzheimer's dementia, Type 2 diabetes, chronic fatigue syndrome, and psychiatric disorders. All of these seem to be occurring at younger and younger ages. There is a great need for tools and strategies that people can use to maximize their body's ability to keep optimal health and vitality.

Research tells us that stress, age, poor diet, and environmental toxins are some of the main culprits that are driving these conditions. All these issues cause inflammation and deplete us of our precious stem cells. Our stem cells are the body's main tools for supporting youth and the ability to heal from injury or disease.

The book you're now reading holds all of Dr. Pompa's best protocols and strategies wrapped up into a seven-week plan. This information is targeted to maximize your body's ability to produce and use new stem cells. Its central premise is to make you highly fat adapted. That way, you are more easily able to take on a five-day water or partial fast during Week 6. Week 6 is where the peak of your body's autophagy and stem cell production occurs. It supplies practical steps each week to prepare you for the fast, plus many adjunctive strategies that increase stem cell activity, stem cell mobilization, and much more.

This whole category of stem cell enhancing strategies that Dr. Pompa has utilized is an excellent adjunct to the emerging field of regenerative medicine. Harnessing the power of stem cells is the future of healthcare. If you relish the idea of shedding stubborn fat, turning back the hands on your biological clock, having more energy, increased brain function, better sleep, and faster recovery, then this book is right up your alley!

ACKNOWLEDGMENTS

My breakthrough for this book occurred because of an exceptional group of people who encouraged me to push through my challenges, understanding that the world needs to know this information. Because of dyslexia, I learned to read much later than most and have struggled with writing. Special thanks to Warren Phillips and Jeff Hayes for consistently providing reliable support and pushing me to get this book done because people need to hear this information.

My wife, Merily, has always been my primary source of inspiration. Beyond her encouragement throughout the writing of this book, she was the one who supported me throughout my unexplainable illness. She ensured me that not only was I going to get well but that I would also share my message with the world. I have to say that her "prophetic" words at that time didn't go over well with me. I told her I couldn't even help myself, let alone help others. That you are holding this book in your hands is a testament to her faith in me.

Merily, hon, thank you for always believing in me. I love you.

This book is only possible through the inspiration and help of many amazing people. I want to take the time to acknowledge all those who contributed.

To Kathryn Kos, you are an answer to our prayers. To edit and make coherent a book a "dyslexic-science mind" like mine wrote is no easy feat. Many have attempted to simplify and make my work more readable without changing the true meaning, and I am left pulling my hair out. Nobody does it better. Thank you.

Cameron George, for providing research. You're one of the smartest guys I know! You are a wealth of knowledge, and I am beyond grateful to you.

Camille, you made up for my greatest weakness of all; providing the recipes and meal plans! The seven-week meal plans are more doable for people because of these resources. Thank you, Camille. I'm sure many will enjoy trying out your delicious recipes.

Diane Hendler, your meticulous help with the final run-through, organization, and finishing touches of this work are greatly appreciated. Thank you, you are an amazing asset, and I look forward to working with you on future projects!

To the HCF (Health Centers of the Future) practitioners who played such a crucial role in the discovery of so much of the content in this book—it is one thing to read a study, but it's another thing to bring it into clinical practice, and sift through what works in real life. I'm proud of you all for being part of a group at the forefront of groundbreaking protocols. Thank you all.

There are so many more who are behind the scenes, including Kathy Gaudry, our amazing editor, and Derek Truninger, our graphic designer. Thank you so much for your hard work to bring this life-changing information to the world. I appreciate your efforts!

Finally, I would also like to thank you, the reader of this book. I hope that this book will change your life, as the information in it has already done for so many others!

INTRODUCTION

Fatigue, low energy, brain fog, weight loss resistance, low libido, anxiety, sleep problems, depression, and other imbalances have become so common today that most people speak of them as being a normal part of aging. Even thyroid dysfunction, diabetes, and other hormone-related conditions are so prevalent that we consider them typical in aging. They may be common, but I can assure you they are not normal. Good news! There is, in fact, a solution to these imbalances. You are holding a science-based solution in your hands right now.

This book goes "beyond fasting" and provides you with daily, monthly, and yearly strategies that for years I have applied to take my health beyond my illness to extraordinary levels in my 50s.

My ultimate passion in life is to empower individuals with information and inspiration from my own "From Pain to Purpose" journey so that you do not fall prey to the avoidable result of chronic disease. From this information, you can expect you will reach your full human potential. After years of struggling with chronic illness, I have rebuilt my health, and so can you.

Since then, I have worked directly with countless sick clients to help them do the same. I've also trained hundreds of doctors in my cellular healing and detoxification protocols. These doctors are known as Health Centers of the Future (HCF) and are located throughout the country and in our network. I've also teamed up with some of the world's most exceptional health professionals, scientists, as well as enthusiasts. Through studying the scientific literature, clinical observation, and self-experimentation, my colleagues and I have come to a strong consensus of which approaches to health and longevity are most effective.

We all agree that the combination of the cellular detox and the strategies you will learn in this book, along with fasting, is how we see people's lives transform and change forever.

This book is a seven-week program with everything I've learned over the years to help people get their lives back and maximize their health and well-being.

This book will take you "beyond fasting" with its expected results for healing the body naturally by leading the reader into the proper preparation for a successful fast. These steps will result in maximum healing and making the fast as easy as possible.

Would you ever run a marathon without training? If you did, your results would not be good. Most likely, you would not finish. It does not differ with doing a fast. This seven-week protocol prepares you for the fast by getting your cells to use their own stored fat as energy (fat adaptation). By going into the fast fat adapted, you will go *Beyond Fasting* because results start Day 1 of the fast. We will lead you to a lifestyle that will change your life forever. It did mine and thousands of others around the world.

Why fast and why is it so transforming? I will build on this answer throughout the book but let me inspire you that fasting has changed my life and millions of other lives. It is the oldest healing therapy known to man used and talked about as far back as the earliest great philosophers, thinkers, and healers for perfect health and as a healing therapy. *Hippocrates, Plato, Socrates, Aristotle, and Galen all used fasting and praised its benefits:*

> **To eat when you are sick is to feed your sickness.**
> —Hippocrates

> **Instead of using medicine, rather, fast a day.**
> —Plutarch

While religious groups may disagree on things such as prayer, one exception is fasting. The spiritual and emotional benefits are real. The Bible doesn't say *if* you fast; it says *when* you fast. I will say that fasting is the most significant reason my wife and I have anti-aged as measured by telomere testing, other tests, and visible physical signs, but the ultimate benefit of all is what it has done for our family.

The *Fasting for a Purpose* Facebook page was born out of God laying on my wife's heart, in the middle of the night, to fast for our son, and all I can tell you is that not only did his life change, but thousands of other lives have changed. Modern science has brought a new understanding to the natural-body miracles that take place with fasting. I trained in fasting in the 90s and just knew it worked for the hardest of all cases, but outside of just knowing the body's innate intelligence (inherent wisdom to heal) caused healing, we could never duplicate it with the best therapies.

We didn't know the science behind the magic. It turns out that stem cells are at the heart of this.

Stem cells are how the body heals and the older we get, the less we have, and the less workable and productive they become for healing. If you cut your arm, stem cells make their way to the injury and form new cells. This healing goes on all day just creating new cells we need to stay healthy, but sickness, toxicity, and age negatively affect our stem cells and affects our healing.

We say the science of stem cells is the future of medicine, and I, too, believe it is, but to date, stem cells are expensive treatments. What if you could fast and get free stem cells? Well, new science says you can. During a fast, the body will use bad cells and debris for energy and nutrition. We call this process, "autophagy." In 2016, Yoshinori Ohsumi, a Japanese scientist, received the Nobel Prize for his discoveries of the mechanisms of autophagy. He says, "Autophagy becomes especially intensive when an organism is under stress, for example, when it fasts. Here, a cell produces energy using its internal resources, cellular rubbish, including pathogenic bacteria."

After the body gets rid of the bad cells through autophagy, which I like to call "Recycle Phase," it stimulates another phase, I call the "Renew Phase." This process is the production of stem cells to replace the cells the body ate for energy and is where the healing happens. Out with the bad and in with the new. The body is amazing. Fasting has even more healing benefits such as hormone optimization, a resetting of gut bacteria and genes, meaning bad genes get turned off, and good genes turned on. Just hold on and welcome the healing and health through fasting and what you are about to learn in this book.

The studies show by Day 5 of a fast we have the highest level of stem cell production. Therefore, we use 5-day fasts to take advantage of this healing. Before I knew the science around this, I found clinically Day 4 people would breakthrough and feel amazing, and the healing would kick in. So, the logic was to go at least four days, but one more day seemed to do the best. Therefore, we did mostly 5-day fasts not knowing there was science around it.

Albert Mosseri (1925-2012), a French researcher, health writer, and advocate of fasting discovered that some people would do well on a partial fast of 500-1000 calories a day and protein under 20 grams a day. Valter Longo, a biogerontologist and cell biologist, has made similar discoveries that autophagy and stem cell production occur during water fasting and he developed the *Fasting Mimicking Diet*™ 5-day meal program that mimics a fasting state. Chapter 6 discusses these various fasting options, including water fast, partial fast, or a *Fasting Mimicking Diet*. This program will help to equip the body with the tools to heal and create new stem cells from Day 1 of the fast, and which rarely happens until Day 4 or 5.

What you learn in the weeks leading up to the fast are the strategies I live my life by whether I am planning to fast or not. This book presents a life guide to better health, not just a plan to maximize your fasting results. Again, the information within the pages of this book goes well *BEYOND FASTING*.

Before you start Week 1, make sure you are available for a five-day fast during Week 6. Look ahead and mark your calendar!

GOING KETO

STARTING FAT ADAPTATION

The goal of this book is to go "beyond fasting" and its expected results for healing the body, naturally. I have created a seven-week program which is being used by doctors around the country with transformative results. The first six weeks of this program will prepare your cells to use fat as their primary energy source—fat adaptation—thereby maximizing the life-changing benefits of fasting. These benefits will go far beyond the fast to a complete lifestyle change that will give you the formula to live a longer and healthier life. You will learn to defy the odds of rapidly increasing degenerative diseases, and the symptoms that have become common in our society such as brain fog, low libido, no energy, anxiety, weight loss resistance, chronic pain, digestive disturbances, the list goes on.

If you didn't read the introduction, go back now so you have an understanding about why fasting and the principles in this book can bring about these changes. Once again, the goal of this program is to reap the maximum healing benefit of a fast starting from Day 1, which rarely happens before Day 4 or 5. For this to occur, complete fat adaptation must happen first.

Here we go! We will start this entire process by introducing you to the *ketogenic* diet, or keto for short. The ketogenic diet is a high fat, moderate protein, low carbohydrate method of eating. Eating this way over a prolonged period puts your body into *ketosis*, a metabolic process in which fat, rather than glycogen, burns as the primary source of fuel. An essential part of this entire plan is eating a low-carbohydrate, high-fat diet. Each week's lesson will build from this plan until we reach our water fast on Week 6. Transitioning to a higher fat, lower carbohydrate diet allows you to start converting your body to burning fat for fuel without restricting calories by eating less.

WHAT IS KETOSIS AND WHAT ARE THE BENEFITS?

Ketosis is a metabolic state characterized by raised levels of ketone bodies. Ketone bodies are compounds produced during the metabolism of fat. Ketosis is a built-in survival mechanism when food or carbohydrates run low.

As a survival mechanism, the body will metabolize fat quickly and make ketones to save your brain. Your brain can only use glucose, or the ketones produced from the breakdown of fat. The brain cannot use fat, so the process is perfect. The body cells can use the fat for energy, and the brain will use the ketones, made from the breakdown of fat when it cannot get glucose. Nutritional ketosis is a healthy state where blood levels of ketones typically range from .5-8.0 milligrams per deciliter (mg/dl).

When you drop your carbohydrate consumption below a certain point, it forces your cells to use fat for energy. Cells can only use two things for energy, sugar or fat, and most people are stuck as sugar burners with the hormonal inability to use fat as energy. To have lasting energy and stay lean in our later years, we need to become more efficient fat burners.

HOW WILL KETOSIS HELP WITH MY FAST DURING WEEK 6?

The key is getting yourself to become more efficient at fat-burning, being fat adapted before the fast begins. This way, you are using the fat stored on and in your body as your energy source from Day 1 of the fast. This use means you feel better during the first few days of the fast when most people feel the worst. Not only do you feel better, but you will also have better results starting from Day 1.

Ketosis triggers the cell renewal process known as autophagy,[1] the recycling phase of the Recycle/Renewal Principle. This process is significant because autophagy will get rid of the old, unwanted cellular materials that struggle to use fat as energy so you can fat adapt faster and make ketones sooner. After the body uses the damaged cells for energy, it raises stem cells to replace them with new, better fat burning cells. The bottom line is if you go into the fast fat adapted, you get more autophagy and therefore produce more stem cells for healing, not to mention feeling better with less unpleasant symptoms.

NUTRITIONAL KETOSIS IN-A-NUTSHELL

Switching from being a sugar-burning metabolizer to becoming a fat-burning metabolizer and producing ketones that have many healing benefits[2] Fat burners stimulate autophagy and new stem cell formation.[3]

Note: Being in a state of nutritional ketosis is safe and differs from diabetic ketoacidosis, a life-threatening complication of diabetes that occurs when the body produces exceedingly elevated levels of ketones in response to a lack of insulin. I recommend working with a trained practitioner when beginning any new diet or health plan.

KETONES ARE A SWITCH FOR YOUR GENES

Back in the early 1900s, we used ketones for seizures,[4] seizure disorders,[5] and many types of neurodegenerative conditions.[6] Ketones have an amazing healing effect on the brain and the cells by reducing inflammation. Aside from reducing cellular inflammation, ketones also turn off bad genes.[7]

The dogma that says you inherited your condition from your mom or dad, and there is nothing you can do about it, is the old science. Genes can be turned on for better or worse, but bad genes or genetic suitability can also be turned off. We call the study of this ability Epigenetics, meaning "above the gene." We see that ketones, or the state of ketosis, turn off bad genes that turned on because of poor lifestyle, toxins, or other stressors. However, when we remove the stressors and apply the principles of this book, we can turn off the bad genes and maximize our health.

The research on ketones over the last five years has been significant and has confirmed in my mind why we all need times of ketosis to live long healthy lives. During ancient times we were forced into these times of ketosis because of the lack of food or types of food that were available (low carb choices like meats and fats). Today most of us must actively choose to take advantage of this survival mechanism that science shows will help us in so many ways.

BENEFITS OF KETONES

 Raise growth hormone and protect all cells and the DNA from oxidative stress.[8]

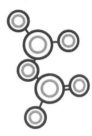

 Reduce inflammation and its markers.[9]

 Protect and repair the mitochondrial membrane and therefore help with fat adaptation.[10]

 Increase cellular energy.[11]

 Burn cleaner metabolically than glucose or fat and therefore create less oxidation and

Turn on the SERT-1 gene that extends life.[13]

For example, research has shown that ketosis provides the following:

- Improved mitochondrial function[14]
- Weight loss[15]
- Mood stabilization[16]
- Hormone regulation[17]
- Turns on genes for longevity (SIRT-1 gene)[18]
- Turns off genes for inflammation[19]
- Re-sets microbiome (gut bacteria), helps good gut bacteria in the gut[20]
- Increased HDL (good) cholesterol[21]
- Lowers triglycerides[22]
- Slows aging[23]
- Blood sugar regulation[24]
- Memory and cognitive improvement[25]
- Neuroprotection (protects our brains from toxins and stress)[26]

Studies also show that ketosis can help certain health conditions, such as:

- Obesity and Hyperlipidemia[27]
- Epilepsy[28]
- Alzheimer's disease[29]
- Parkinson's disease[30]
- Cancer[30]
- Acne[32]
- Polycystic ovary syndrome (PCOS)[33]
- Cardiovascular disease[34]
- Autism[35]
- Metabolic syndrome[36]
- Fatty liver disease[37]

KETONES AND YOUR GUT

Ketones help to heal the gut and help to diversify the gut microbiome.[38] Ketones burn exceptionally clean, like natural gas on a stove. This process helps to down-regulate inflammation. I could go on and on about the benefits of ketones, but I will focus on a big one. If you are fearful about the Week 6 fast, ketosis makes it so much easier and tolerable.

When you go into a fasted state already in ketosis, you won't have that three- day adjustment period of your body wanting to reach for carbohydrates as the source of fuel. The body will already reach for fat and will at once burn fat for fuel. This change makes fasting much less of a struggle in terms of hunger and cravings.

HOW DO I GET INTO KETOSIS AND BECOME FAT ADAPTED?

It typically takes two to four weeks to become fat adapted, or in full ketosis. For most people, it will happen in two weeks. For some people, it can even happen in one week. It isn't a complicated, lengthy process for most people. Do not overthink it. Limit your carbohydrate consumption to under 50 grams per day and be careful with protein intake. This plan differs from the low carbohydrate Atkins™ diet. Don't worry about much else; focus on limiting carbs at first. Make the carbs you are consuming come from vegetable sources, rather than grains which can drive inflammation. Most people will transition into ketosis by keeping carbohydrates under 50 grams per day. However, people with more significant metabolic issues need to drop to 30 grams or fewer to enter ketosis.

How can you tell if your body is in ketosis? The presence of ketones in your body is proof you're in ketosis. The best method to test for ketones is using a blood meter, which is much more accurate than urine testing. Urine testing is not as effective because ketones will rise in urine in just a few days, but all it means is that you are making ketones, not that you are using them. After you become adapted in a few weeks, the urine ketones drop as an indicator you are using the ketones. This drop causes people to become confused, so don't spend your time using the urine strips.

I recommend using blood ketone meters, such as Keto-Mojo, which can measure your blood sugar and blood ketones. You will need to buy ketone testing strips separately from the meter. Both are available on their site at www.getketomojo.com.

When testing, if blood ketones measure between .5 and 8.0, you're in ketosis, as the average range is between 1.0 and 3.0. When you are fasting, you will typically see numbers between 3.0–9.0. I prefer the Keto- Mojo because the strips for ketones are only $1.00 each as opposed to other meter strips that can be as high as $4.00 a strip.

It's fun to watch your body go through this transition, gradually making more ketones, and becoming fat adapted. Typically, the first week your ketones will register below .5 or even say "low" but will slowly rise. Be patient; for most, it takes two to three weeks to fat-adapt and get into ketosis. Some will find it takes more time, so you may even need to lower your carbs or protein intake.

WORDS OF ADVICE FOR THOSE OF YOU TRACKING KETONE LEVELS

Don't use urine ketone strips for accurate ketone measurements. Your body is now using your ketones, so they won't show in the urine. You may notice ketones in your urine in the beginning, but recall, your brain starts using them, so you don't want to keep seeing them in your urine as you progress through the fast.

Ketones circulating in the blood may climb up higher in a few weeks after you first fat adapt, but then lower some as you are using them in your body. Breath ketones can be useful because it shows the oxidized ketones or ketones you are using. However, because there is a delay, it is difficult to assess which foods are doing what to your ketone production.

Therefore, we use the blood ketones as the fastest and most exact way to determine ketosis, determining max autophagy, and fasting windows during intermittent fasting, which is something about which you will learn.

WHAT IF I AM NOT IN KETOSIS OR
LOSING FAT AFTER A FEW WEEKS?

For those of you who have health challenges and toxicity issues, it may take a fasting state (Week 6 of this program) for your ketones to go up and stay up. Keep at it and don't give up. Later in the book, I talk about diet variation (feast/famine cycles) as a cellular biohack for those who struggle to breakthrough to fat adaptation. Toxicity plays a significant role here. Some of you may be neurotoxic and may have hormonally lost the ability to use fat efficiently in your mitochondria. My cellular detoxification work has become an answer for so many who have tried it all and wonder what is wrong because they eat better than everyone and yet still can't burn fat. Hang in there—the answer is coming!

My cellular detox program is the game changer for many, but I will say that it's not just one fast, but multiple fasts and even daily and weekly fasting, which you will learn in the coming chapters, that are my main strategies. Make fasting a lifestyle choice and watch your life change for the better. My wife and I have practiced these principles for years, and we will both tell you that every year our health and metabolic flexibility (our ability to move in and out of ketosis and burn fat) has increased. We can be out of ketosis for months and in days move right back in. It took time to get here, especially for my wife, but now we are leaner and healthier in our fifties than we were in our twenties.

"My husband always says that skinny people who have trouble using fat for energy, store their fat in their organs. This, would be even more problematic, and something I wanted to be sure to correct."[39]

Being in a state of ketosis helps you to live longer. This goal has become more important for my wife and me, as we see our five children becoming adults. I have two goals that drive me. One is the fear of getting sick again—I can't ever go back there. Two, I want to not just be around for my grandkids, but to ski and bike and do the things I love to do with them. For me, it is not as much about living longer as it is about being healthy longer. If I can't enjoy life, why live longer?

IT ALL SOUNDS AMAZING BUT
WHAT DO I DO WITH MY CRAVINGS?

When you become a fat burner, the body releases cholecystokinin, which stimulates the gallbladder to release bile.[40] This helps to decrease cravings and appetite, because you will digest and better assimilate these healthy fats.

Cholecystokinin also reduces appetite by turning off the appetite mechanism.

A hormone called ghrelin controls appetite, and cholecystokinin influences this hormone and causes you to feel satisfied.[41,42] Even before you become fat adapted by eating more fat in your diet, you will release more cholecystokinin and reduce hunger as well. So, load up on good fats as described below, but when you first start, you may need a digestive enzyme that has ox bile (bile salts) and lipase.

WHAT ABOUT PROTEIN INTAKE?

Many people mistake ketosis for the Atkins™ Diet and load up on proteins, such as meat, to replace the reduced carbohydrates.[43] We want to consume moderate amounts of protein since protein converts to glucose through a process called gluconeogenesis. Research reveals that too much protein consumption for an extended amount of time stimulates a pathway called the mTOR pathway linked to premature aging and health problems.44 However, short periods of increased protein intake, which stimulates mTOR, can be beneficial. We will discuss this later.

Consume half of your (lean) body weight in protein. For a 150-pound person, stay around 75 grams of protein per day, and under 50 for carbs. If you are highly active and work out, you could go up to 75% of your lean body weight. That's 100 grams for the 150-pound person. It's that simple. Try not to overcomplicate from here. You must wonder, what can I eat?

THE FAT DIFFERENCE

As you decrease carbohydrates and protein in your diet, with what do you replace them? Fat! Don't panic; fat does not make you fat.[45] That's an old myth disproven so many times over the last twenty years. But while it may be old news, it's true; fat doesn't make you fat. It helps you become a more efficient fat burner.

To ensure you replace your lost calories with quality fat calories, and since we don't restrict calories, I have developed my 2-2-2-2 rule. This rule will make sure you consume enough fat and a variety of quality fat. The amount will also help ward off what is known as *keto flu*—symptoms some experience the first week of ketosis, which can feel like the flu.

Let me introduce my **KETOGENIC** 2-2-2-2 **RULE -** The heart of ketosis:

 2 tablespoons of coconut or MCT oil (a fat supplement made of medium-chain triglycerides). You can eat it right off a spoon, or put it in a smoothie or shake, or even cook with it. The medium chain triglycerides help you to burn fat, and help with suppressing the appetite as well.

CAUTION: Too much MCT or even coconut oil all at once can cause stomach upset, so better to spread it out.

2 tablespoons grass-fed butter or ghee, off the spoon or cook with it. This gives you healthy saturated fats to help with energy and stabilizing the appetite.

 2 tablespoons olive oil, avocado oil, or macadamia nut oil. This gives you healthy monounsaturated fats, and we are mixing up the fats (which is good to do). Avocado oil is also great for cooking at high temperatures. Another option is to get healthy non-denature omega 6 and 3 such as Andreas Seed Oils (andreasseedoil.com). They are true cold-pressed oils like sunflower or pumpkin seed oil that would normally oxidized during processing. These oils high in omega 6 are needed in your cell membranes. This is important for many health conditions.

2 teaspoons sea salt. When you start fat-adapting, you will lose stored sugar from your muscles and your gycogen. This will cause the loss of some water and therefore electrolytes. The sea salt can help with feeling weak or dizzy, and help you through the adjustment period of becoming fat-adapted. This makes a big difference with the 'keto flu'.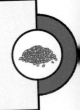

WHAT CAN I EAT ON A KETOGENIC DIET?

Here are some foods acceptable on a ketogenic diet:

 Raw hard cheeses (as tolerated, organic).

 Eggs

 A variety of nuts, preferably activated (which means soaked and then dehydrated. This ensures they are easier to

 Berries (have a low glycemic index, and can be consumed moderation).

 Grass-fed steak, lamb, chicken, turkey... essentially all animal-based protein sources are ketogenic friendly. You don't want to overdo protein, so opting for the fattier cuts is a good way to make sure you're getting enough fat with the protein. Opt for organic, grass-fed meat to ensure it does not contain any added hormones, antibiotics, and is also as nutrient dense as

 Organ meats (organic, pasture-raised) are also an extremely good choice, and are more nutrient dense than other conventional cuts of meat

 Prepared/cured meats (like salami and sausage) are OK so long as they are organic, grass-fed, don't have any added sugars and are preservative and nitrate free.

 Healthy fats 2/2/2 rule (2 tablespoons MCT or coconut oil, 2 tablespoons grass-fed butter or ghee, 2 tablespoons olive oil, macadamia nut oil, or avocado oil.

 Smoothies

To fully understand the principles of a ketogenic diet, know that all calories are not created equal and that not all macronutrients are created equal either. Calories-in-calories-out style diets are heavily disproven by modern science,[47] which gives way to the ketogenic diet as a means of eating without ever having to count calories.[48] Your focus is on the foods you eat, which is a diet high in fats, moderate in protein, and low in carbohydrates.

Ketone bodies, or ketones, are by-products of the body breaking down fat for energy when carbohydrate intake is low. On a higher carbohydrate diet, the body runs on glucose or sugar, but on a low-carb ketogenic diet, the body runs effectively on ketones or fat.

UNDERSTANDING CARB COUNTING

Although we want to keep our carbohydrate consumption to under 50 grams per day, we are shooting for net carbs, meaning you minus the fiber from this equation. Let's say you determine your food has 10 grams of carbs and 5 grams are from fiber, then your net carbs are 5 grams. There are many vegetables you can eat once you minus the fiber and the net carbs are lower.

There is a free app called *Cronometer*, which is a comprehensive nutrition tracker that breaks down nutrients tracking how much fat, protein, and carbohydrates you are consuming each day. After a few days of tracking, you will catch on, and may not need to track further. Although some find it helpful to keep track of everything, it isn't necessary for the long term. Google is another great tool. Google, "How many carbs in a cup of berries?" and you will get your answer.

CAN YOU HAVE LEGUMES AND LENTILS?

Yes, legumes and lentils are okay to consume, but track the net carbs on them. You will probably need to eat less of these than usual, as they are carb heavy. The same rule applies to ancient grains such as Quinoa. Watch the carbs. Stay under the 50 grams, and you will be golden.

When consuming legumes, make sure you soak (and sprout) them before consuming. Soak them in filtered water overnight, and then rinse properly before cooking, and this will dispose of most of the lectins which make them hard for your body to digest.

UNDERSTANDING THE KETO FLU

When you become an efficient fat burner, your body releases many accumulated toxins that exist in the fat stores. As toxins circulate throughout the bloodstream, they can bring about many negative symptoms until processed and excreted by your system.

These symptoms are temporary and usually clear up within a few days. An electrolyte imbalance can also cause keto flu. The two teaspoons of sea salt from my 2-2-2-2 rule each day will help you. The sea salt will help balance your electrolytes, and you'll begin to feel better. It's also vital to stay hydrated. So, drink plenty of water.

THREE REASONS YOU MIGHT NOT FEEL WELL AND SOME SOLUTIONS

1. **Low electrolytes:** Add sea salt to your water to help maintain electrolytes. Taking magnesium may help some—I recommend magnesium malate or magnesium glycinate. Or, you may need to take a stronger, more balanced electrolyte; find one without sugar.

2. **Not be fully fat adapted:** You may need to spend more time in the earlier steps or more variation in the diet weekly or monthly (see Weeks 4 and 5).

3. **Still not fat adapted even following this protocol?** You may be struggling with some neurotoxicity. I recommend our "fasting trio" CytoDetox®, BIND, and Fastonic. However, some may have deep toxic issues and need one of our Platinum doctors trained in Cellular Detox.

- **Fastonic** down-regulates hydroxy free radicals. Free radicals cause inflammation and unwanted symptoms, especially during fasting.

- **BIND** prevents the toxins from the gut recirculating back into the body, called auto-intoxication, which leads to many unwanted symptoms.

- **CytoDetox®** helps support the body in the toxin elimination from the cells.

The drop in glucose that occurs is another factor that contributes to the keto flu. The cells are still in "sugar burning"' mode. However, as fat and keto-adaptation happen, you will feel better quickly. It takes a few weeks to adapt. Even when you produce ketones, it doesn't mean your brain is using them efficiently yet. Therefore, the brain can still feel a little off. I can always tell when I am keto-adapted because I feel like I can think circles around everyone, and my memory improves drastically. Regardless, you *will* get through this period, typically only a couple of days for most people, especially if the struggle is because of electrolytes.

I am encouraging you to trek through. Going through this short rough period will set you up for long-term success. The cravings will go away once you become fat adapted, and your energy will also increase. Here is a seven-day sample meal plan to help. The recipes in the *Meal Plans and Recipes* section are italicized.

A SEVEN-DAY SAMPLE MEAL PLAN TO HELP
GET YOU THROUGH THIS WEEK

NOTE: Italicized items can be found in the *Meal Plans and Recipes* section.

Monday—Day One Breakfast: *Chia Pudding*

    Snack: Handful of macadamia nuts

    Lunch: Raw vegetables, red pepper dip, baba ghanoush, and some

    Liver Pâté

    Dinner: Steak with grilled asparagus, avocado, and charred jalapeños

Tuesday—Day Two

    Breakfast: Green Berry Smoothie

    Snack: Carrots, celery, and Guacamole

    Lunch: Leftover steak with grilled asparagus, avocado, charred jalapeños

    Dinner: Eggplant Parmesan

Wednesday—Day Three

    Breakfast: Creamy Chocolate Avocado Smoothie

    Snack: Collagen Cookie Dough Balls

    Lunch: Grilled fish with cucumber, feta, tomato, and olive salad

    Dinner: Chicken Zoodle Soup

Thursday—Day Four

    Breakfast: Loaded Mexican-style *Omelet* with shredded chicken, cheese, chives, parsley, coriander, salsa, and sour cream

    Snack: Two hard-boiled eggs

    Lunch: Sashimi with seaweed salad

    Dinner: *Roast Chicken* with *Cauliflower Mash*

Friday—Day Five

Breakfast: Poached eggs on a bed of arugula, with grilled asparagus, avocado, and mushrooms

Snack: A spoonful of almond butter and a handful of berries

Lunch: Leftover *Roast Chicken* with *Spicy Turmeric Roasted Cauliflower*

Dinner: *Zucchini Noodles with Pesto* and *Beef Meatballs*

Saturday—Day Six

Breakfast: Chia Pudding

Snack: Green Berry Smoothie

Lunch: Beef Tataki with an Asian style slaw

Dinner: Cauliflower Crust Pizza topped with pesto, chicken and arugula

Sunday—Day Seven

Breakfast: Chocolate Avocado Pudding

Snack: Handful of Brazil nuts

Lunch: Leftover Cauliflower Crust Pizza topped with pesto, chicken and arugula

Dinner: Oven-baked salmon with roasted fennel and carrots

KETO CONVENIENCE FOODS

Canned sardines, oysters, sock-eye salmon, mackerel, anchovies, or sardines (in olive oil and sea salt), raw macadamia nuts, roasted nori seaweed snacks, hard-boiled or deviled eggs, raw coconut butter, avocados, homemade fat bombs, grass-fed cheese/yogurt, guacamole with EPIC pastured pork rinds or bacon chips, sugar-free jerky, high-fat smoothies and puddings, homemade unsweetened popsicle, grass-fed whey protein powders, Bulletproof and EPIC bars.

TROUBLESHOOTING: COMMON BEGINNER MISTAKES

Many people eagerly begin the ketogenic diet but give up shortly after that for lack of results. I've seen these common mistakes to avoid for keto success:

- **Excess protein consumption** - Beware of gluconeogenesis, where excess protein converts to sugar and stores as fat.

- **Excess caloric intake -** Strategic calorie restriction and intermittent fasting is key and discussed in later chapters.

- **You are not consuming enough healthy dietary fat -** If you consume enough fat, you shouldn't feel uncomfortable hunger or cravings.

- **Not accounting for all carbs -** Food journaling can supply accountability.

- **Too much, or too little physical activity -** Properly timed burst training is best for rapid fat-loss and hormone optimization.

- **Electrolyte loss -** The 2-2-2-2 Rule is vital here.

A WORD ON EXOGENOUS KETONES

Some companies are selling human-made ketone supplements. These can be helpful for athletes and those who are looking to boost their mental performance and struggling to get into ketosis. The verdict is still out on long-term use, but they have a place as a beneficial, supportive tool. Bottom line: Supplemental ketones are a shortcut to experiencing the feeling of ketosis, a gift from science. However, for the "real deal" ketosis, cells must be trained naturally to burn the body's fat for energy, which takes time and effort.

EATING LESS OFTEN

HOW MANY TIMES DO YOU EAT EACH DAY?

Most Americans today are in a constant state of feeding.[1] People see themselves as eating two to three meals a day, but for most people, it's much more than that. That handful of nuts you eat when you walk through the kitchen? That is a meal. The kombucha you chugged? That is a meal. Anything that stimulates glucose or insulin is doing the same thing in the body—forcing digestion.

The studies show that people who eat less live longer.[2] However, when looking at ancient cultures, people ate less by *eating less often*, fewer meals. Eating less does not mean eating half of your food and pushing the rest aside. That would be a calorie-restricted diet, which, unfortunately, is the accepted core concept of weight loss, even by medical professionals. You cannot read an article or watch a television program about weight loss without hearing about reducing your calories to lose weight. The media is always pushing the next low-fat and low-calorie recipe and diets. If it were only so easy.[3]

Every time you reduce calories to lose weight, your metabolism slows.[4] At first, you will lose some weight, which leads us to the notion that caloric restriction does, in fact, work. The problem is that you may lose some weight initially, but the fat-burning stops as a survival mechanism the body uses to hold on to the precious fuel it needs because food is getting scarce. If the body thinks it is starving, it will hold on to the fat at all cost despite your efforts to go lower and lower on daily calories consumed. Even if you are super disciplined, you could find yourself eating 500 calories a day, not losing weight, and wondering why.

On average, with the strictest low-calorie diet, women may lose 10–15 pounds and men 15–20 pounds, but the weight loss will stop as the body retains its stored energy, fat. There is no long-term success with caloric restriction, and the science shows this. However, some still acknowledge it as being an answer. Poor results leave us feeling as though it's our fault, or we are doing something wrong. Worse yet, it makes us feel guilty of being perceived as lazy, lacking in exercise, or gluttonous and overeating.

Hormones are the key to weight loss and lasting energy, but it is optimizing hormones, not taking them, along with the strategies in this book that holds and proves to be the genuine answer.[5]

Even not being able to control cravings and sticking to a healthy diet is more about hormones than discipline. Trust me; it is not your fault. It is your hormones.

The first lesson we can gain by emulating ancient cultures to perfect our hormones is to eat less by eating less often. This strategy goes far beyond weight loss. The studies are correct; to live healthy longer, we must eat less. Eating less, by eating less often, raises growth hormone[6] and allows our cells to hear the hormone signals better (hormone optimization), preventing the body from going into the survival mechanism for starvation. The hormone changes also improve our health and longevity.[7] This is a win/win situation!

The Biosphere 2 Project proved that caloric restriction by merely eating less does not work. After insect and animal studies showed that a 25–30% decrease in daily caloric intake extended life, the project used human subjects. Seven human subjects lived in a pristine biosphere for two years in a 25-30% caloric restricted plant-based diet. It was a complete failure as specific longevity genes turned on as expected, but their organs shrank, and their immune systems suffered. They went into a catabolic state, which can include extreme fatigue, joint and muscle pain, and sleeplessness, that could not support a healthy lifestyle.

One lesson that scientist Valter Longo, creator of the Fasting Mimicking Diet which we discuss later in this book, learned from this project was that long-term caloric restriction does not work, but short periods, such as five days a month, the core of his diet system, works.

The most important lesson is that eating less with caloric restriction fails overall because the body goes into a starvation mode, but eating less by eating less often optimizes the body hormonally, preventing starvation and muscle loss.

You will live longer healthy and stay lean your whole life by eating less often. It is essential to recognize that the opposite is also true. Eating five or six meals a day can increase your risk of developing chronic disease.[8] I love to say that if you want to die sooner with more disease, eat more often.

Begin by cutting down the number of times you eat per day to three times. Cut out all snacks and consume just three meals. It may sound easy until you realize how many times a day you walk by the kitchen and eat a few berries or nuts. Adopt a new rule of consuming only three meals during this week—that is it!

We intend Week 2 to take your fat adaptation to the next level. You are already following a ketogenic diet. Now we are reducing the number of times you eat a day, which is slowly getting your body more used to burning its fat for energy.

A FEW SIMPLE STEPS YOU CAN TAKE THIS WEEK IN PREPARATION

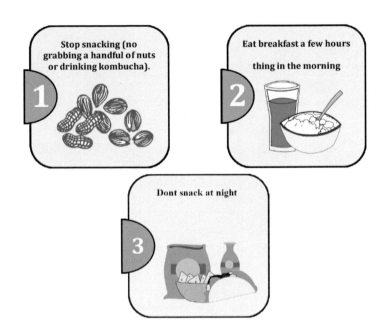

During this second week, the body will increase ketone production. If you burn sugar as your primary fuel, you may struggle with headaches or irritability between meals. Don't fret; this goes away in time and will prepare you for fasting.

I CANNOT GO WITHOUT SNACKS

In my practice, I often hear from clients, "I am hypoglycemic, and therefore, I have to eat snacks during the day, or I will have no energy." Clients often claim they will get dizzy or even pass out if they don't snack often enough. Without meals or snacks every few hours, many people experience symptoms such as irritability, feeling 'hangry,' dizzy, and having headaches. My typical response is, "Yes, I know and expect this to be difficult, but it is critically important for you to regain your health."

When I instruct people, I call this method of missing meals and snacks *metabolic mitochondrial fitness*. This term means that with the added stress of going without food, the cells will become more efficient fat burners.[9] For example, those who never, or rarely exercise will typically feel worse in the beginning before adjusting to the new movements. Once fat adaptation occurs, you begin to not only feel better but become healthier. The mitochondria produce energy from within, and when the mitochondria become more efficient at using fat for energy, we can go longer and longer periods without food, yet have lasting energy and singular focus. I like to say you are now *fat adapted* or *metabolically flexible.* If glucose is present, you will burn it,[10] but if it is not available, you will burn your fat for energy.

Cells can only use two things for energy: sugar (carbohydrates) or fat.[11] Healthy people with healthy cells can use both when needed. I consider these people metabolically flexible. For example, If you are not eating, the cells will get energy from your stored fat and have a stable constant energy supply, meaning no lightheadedness or symptoms from the lack of food.

Today most people have lost their ability to use fat as an energy source efficiently. These are the people I refer to as sugar burners. If you are stuck as a sugar burner and cannot yet use fat for energy, you may notice a sudden drop in energy, to the point of feeling very weak and lifeless. Even the brain stops the best functioning because it's just not getting the glucose it needs. We call this brain fog, and many people struggle with this today because of cellular inability to use fat as energy.

Being stuck as a sugar burner leads to hypoglycemia and hormone dysregulation, weight loss resistance, fatty liver, diabetes, thyroid conditions, and the list goes on.[12] Hypoglycemia is a prelude to many of these conditions. The answer is simple: Get the cells (mitochondria) to burn fat, especially when not eating.

Just like with a new exercise regimen, your cells will adapt and become better and better at using fat, but you will need to go through some days or weeks of not feeling great to become an efficient fat burner. When you achieve this fat-adapted state, you will also find you lose the cravings for carbs and sugar and have lasting energy all day despite not eating.

SOME WORDS OF ENCOURAGEMENT

Before finding the *Beyond Fasting* solution, my wife Merily needed to eat all day. I knew her to eat huge meals, and I recall commenting one day that she eats like a linebacker. I can assure you she did not look like one. She was the perfect weight for her body type. However, if we do not store fat on our body, it will store in our organs like the liver or pancreas, leading to other diseases and problems. Therefore, regardless of our weight, we are all at risk of experiencing health issues if we are sugar-burning metabolizers.

WHAT IS HAPPENING IN THE BODY DURING WEEK 2?

How does cutting down on meals increase stem cells? When your body is fasting, not digesting as often, the body will eat the decrepit tissue.[13,14] The body knows to eat the bad cells before the functional cells. This process is autophagy! Then the body stimulates new stem cell formation to replace the bad cells it's used for energy. The new cells are healthy and able to burn fat more efficiently. The more we practice going without food and experience mitochondrial metabolic fitness, the more lasting energy we have, the leaner we become, and the younger we look.

WHAT IF YOU DON'T WANT TO LOSE WEIGHT?

Although you may lose weight, this is not a weight loss focused program. The focus of this program is towards the destruction of harmful cells, and new stem cell formation. We are turning back the years on aging and fighting off inflammatory conditions.

My son was at about 3% body fat and wanting to put muscle on. He wanted to start a water fast. However, he worried that with fasting, he would lose muscle and lose weight. I told him he might lose some weight, but to watch what happens a month after the fast. After fasting, he gained ten pounds of muscle. Over months my son put on even more muscle. Why is this?

Some substandard tissue, proteins that the body uses for energy, healing, and repair, get replaced with new proteins via stem cells.[15] These are healthy cells, with a better ability to recover, and therefore, the new muscle grows. Stem cells can form new proteins in joints, organs, or whatever else needs healing and repair.[16] Therefore, my doctors and I use fasting as a tool to help those who need to gain healthy weight, not just lose unwanted fat.

THE BOTTOM LINE

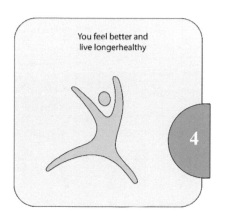

Less meals/ snacking = Autophagy !
Your body will start to eat the bad tissues, and stimulate stem cells to replece the bad cells

1

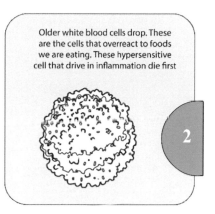

Older white blood cells drop. These are the cells that overreact to foods we are eating. These hypersensitive cell that drive in inflammation die first

2

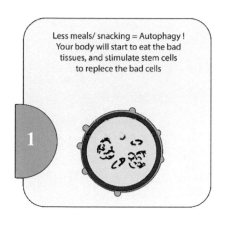

You feel better and live longerhealthy

4

3

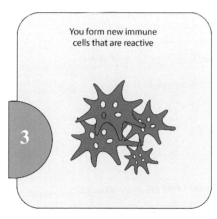

You form new immune cells that are reactive

You are taking the next step to becoming an efficient fat burner by cutting down on the number of times you eat during the day. This change will prepare your body for the next step of intermittent fasting, where you eat even less often, in a small window. Week by week, we are slowly turning your body into a fat-burning machine, which again burns cleaner and down-regulates inflammation. This process will be easier than you think.

REMEMBER: DON'T EAT LESS. EAT LESS OFTEN.

- To live longer and healthier.
- To hormonally optimize to a metabolically efficient fat burner.
- To shut down hyperimmunity and feel and think better.

WEEK 2 SAMPLE MEAL PLAN

NOTE: Italicized items can be found in the *Meal Plans and Recipes* section.

Monday—Day One

Breakfast: Poached eggs on a bed of arugula, grilled mushrooms, and avocado

Lunch: Grilled fish with cucumber, feta, tomato, and olive salad

Dinner: *Roast Chicken* with charred broccoli and *Spicy Turmeric Roasted Cauliflower*

Tuesday—Day Two

Breakfast: *Chia Pudding* with cinnamon, blueberries, chopped nuts

Lunch: Nori rolls with sardines, cucumber, sprouts, and peppers

Dinner: Baked potato loaded with pulled chicken, bacon, cheese, chives, and sour cream

Wednesday—Day Three

Breakfast: Breakfast frittata with roasted red peppers, spinach, and feta

Lunch: *Roasted Vegetables Drizzled with Olive Oil and Sea Salt*, salad with arugula, drizzled with avocado oil

Dinner: Steak with grilled asparagus, avocado, and charred jalapeños

Thursday—Day Four

Breakfast: *Chocolate Avocado Pudding*

Lunch: BBQ'd chicken with grilled eggplant and zucchini drizzled with
Lemon Tahini Sauce

Dinner: Lamb with roasted carrots and salad

Friday—Day Five

Breakfast: Yogurt or kefir with berries and granola and nuts

Lunch: Chicken Pad Thai with Shirataki noodles

Dinner: *Cauliflower Crust Pizza* topped with pesto, chicken, and arugula

Saturday—Day Six

Breakfast: *Strawberry Mint Smoothie*

Lunch: Mushroom soup topped with seeds and avocado

Dinner: *Beef Mushroom Lettuce Tacos*

Sunday—Day Seven

Breakfast: *Chia Pudding*

Lunch: *Green Soup* with avocado, toasted seeds, and olive oil

Dinner: *Chicken Zoodle Soup*

INTERMITTENT FASTING
AND THE EATING WINDOW

Notice the title of this week is "The Eating Window" not "The Starving Window." One principle for this week is eating until you are full. That sounds much better. However, this still involves fasting but for a much shorter time, typically for fifteen to twenty-four hours. Studies show that even short fasts like this produce autophagy and therefore, some stem cells rise.[1] Not as much as you would get with a more extended block fast, but when you fast daily, or several times per week, the benefits are significant and noticed.

I think a better way to understand intermittent daily fasting, is to think of specific eating windows, such as a four, six, or eight-hour window. For sample eating window times, reference the graphic below.

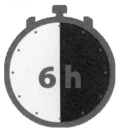  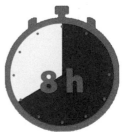

One example is to eat two meals within the six-hour window. This schedule creates a more extended fasting period and higher autophagy. The body is eating the bad stuff, and we get a rise in stem cells, and this is when the magic happens. Darn easy for some of you at this point because you're in ketosis.

HOW AND WHY DOES THIS MAKE MY FAST EASIER AND MAXIMIZE MY STEM CELLS?

Once again, it all boils down to forcing fat adaptation and autophagy, to drive up the stem cells. By the time you start your fast, you can receive the benefits on Day 1. Intermittent fasting, which is more than ketosis and an extended block fast forces the body to adapt to having no food and burning fat for energy. The adaptation makes the cells more efficient at using fat for energy, and autophagy eats the bad cells and cellular rubbish first before using functional cells.[2] Your body wants to and knows how to survive. The moment these adaptations start, the stem cells rise, and so do the benefits. Three fundamental diet changes drive autophagy. Intermittent fasting can potentially take advantage of all three.

THE THREE DIET CHANGES THAT DRIVE AUTOPHAGY

- No-calories fasting/Low-calories partial fast/or Fasting Mimicking Diet - The best way to eat less is by eating less often. Intermittent fasting, by eating one to two meals in a small window, is the best way to eat fewer calories or no calories without slowing your metabolism, and to trigger autophagy.

- Low protein to moderate protein - When skipping meals, your protein intake automatically drops and by intentionally eating less than 15–20 grams a day of protein, you can really drive autophagy.[3]

- Low carbohydrates - Like low protein, if you skip meals when your carbohydrates drop, autophagy occurs.

Daily intermittent fasting (IF) is by far the best thing my wife and I have done for our health in our wiser years. My cellular detoxification saved our lives, but intermittent fasting took them to another level of fitness, leanness, and energy. It is one of the most effective tools I have used for hormone optimization. We both noticed an anti-aging effect as over time the body gets better at using fat for energy when you are not eating, the metabolic flexibility I referred to earlier. Although the autophagy is less than you would get in a block fast, it occurs daily, and the benefits accumulate with time.[4] We are both getting older but leaner and healthier each year.

In the earlier chapters, I mentioned that the real issue with weight loss is not how much we are eating or exercising; it's our hormones. If we want to optimize our hormones, we must get our cells to hear our hormones, rather than taking exogenous hormones. Although there is also a time and a place to take exogenous hormones, the biggest issue is not the lack of hormones. The cells cannot communicate with our hormones effectively. Fasting increases the cells' ability to hear the hormones. A hormone must attach to a receptor on the cell and relay the message to the cell for the hormone to communicate with it. Here, we are telling the cell to burn fat as energy.

Intermittent fasting will also achieve hormone optimization by increasing growth hormone and other hormones needed for weight loss and make our cells more sensitive to our hormone. There is a scientific study showing that during fasted states, we increase growth hormone to prevent muscle loss as part of autophagy.[5]

Many studies are showing an increase in insulin sensitivity, even on short daily fasting. Insulin is the fat-storing hormone, and a huge reason people are sick and can't lose weight. Getting your cells to hear and be more sensitive to insulin is a massive part of why intermittent fasting has so much anti-aging power.[6] As we fast, this occurs not just with insulin but all hormones. The more fasting you practice, the healthier and leaner you become. However, as I stated, it takes time. If I can get you to make this a lifestyle, and not another fad diet you move in and out of, I know your life will profoundly change forever.

Living longer with health and vitality is one of my goals, and at the forefront of the studies is a caloric restriction. Just trying to cut calories may work for life extension in a lab, but not long-term health and even weight loss. After studying ancient cultures, I've concluded that the way to eat less and live long is to be eating less often.

You can't argue with the studies on eating less and life extension.[7] There are many reasons why this extends life. First, eating less by eating less often extends something known as *telomeres* at the end of our chromosomes. Telomeres are the only biological clock we know. The shorter they get, the closer we come to death. Picture the little plastic piece on the end of your shoelace, protecting the lace. That is the telomere at the end of your chromosomes. The shorter it gets, the closer you are to dying. Intermittent fasting lengthens the telomere which studies associated with living longer. You can measure your telomeres. Mine have dramatically gotten better and better through my cellular detox program and fasting.

There are other things you can do to lengthen your telomeres like take TA 65, a drug shown in past animal studies, and now statistically in a 2016 study with humans,[8] to lengthen telomeres.[9] However, fasting has more research behind it and is a less expensive option.

The second way to increase telomeres is eating less. By eating less often, you are extending your life by increasing something known as the NAD+/ NADH ratio. The higher the NAD+ compared to the NADH, the longer you might live. A high NAD+/NADH ratio identifies a marker for caloric restriction. Increasing the ratio allows gene expression changes that lead to increased life spans in animals.[10] It's important to note that calorie restriction has many benefits other than just increased lifespan.

In animals, it has been shown that fasting reduces the incidence of age- related diseases such as Alzheimer's, Parkinson's disease, Type 2 diabetes, cardiovascular disease, autoimmune disease, and even cancer. While these are animal studies and may or may not translate to humans, I can tell you that after years of studying fasting in humans; we see the same results.[11]

Many of us are eating certain foods that help raise NAD+ and even doing NAD+ intravenously. I have done the NAD+ IV's, and while I felt a boost of energy, fasting is more effective and less expensive.

Another method of raising the NAD+/NADH ratio that appears to invoke a restricted caloric state and extend life is taking something known as "oxaloacetate."[12]

Supplemental oxaloacetate enters the cell and breaks down into malate,[13] and in that breakdown, NADH converts to NAD+. In animal models, oxaloacetate supplementation increases both NAD+ levels and the NAD+/NADH ratio, inducing a caloric-reduced state and increasing their lifespan.[14] Fasting is by far the most effective, most studied and least expensive way of not just extending life via telomeres or NAD+/NADH ratio, but also reducing your chances of age-related diseases that are affecting so many at an alarming rate.

Every thriving culture has done intermittent fasting. We are just not forced to do so in our culture. The first time I experienced this way of eating was in Africa, and I didn't know what to make of it. At that time, I was still a believer in four to six meals a day to support muscle and lose fat. I saw the men leave for long daily hunts on foot early in the morning and return late afternoon without eating breakfast or lunch—they ate one big meal a day. It lasted three hours, like in European countries, but it was a feast that would tell their body it is far from starving, unlike caloric restriction. There were no diseases as in other tribes, and they had recently come out of the mountains because of drought, so they still practiced most of their traditional ways of living. These people are living long and healthy lives.

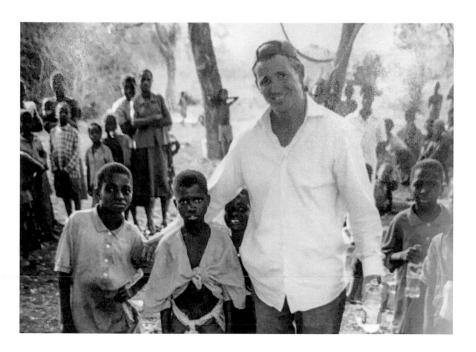

If you want to live a long healthy life, don't eat less, eat less often. Studies on the number of meals a day show the more meals, the worse the results for long-term health and weight loss.[15]

A recent study released in the September 6, 2018 issue of *Cell Metabolism* proves my point well.[16] The mice who ate once a day lived up to 40 percent longer than the ones that had access to food around the clock. According to NIA Director Richard Hodes, MD, "This study showed that mice who ate one meal per day, and thus had the longest fasting period, seemed to have a longer lifespan and better outcomes for common age- related liver disease and metabolic disorders."[17]

THE SPECIFICS ON "HOW TO"

Although it may sound complicated, intermittent fasting is a straight-forward concept. It's eating in a four to six, maybe eight-hour window. Perhaps you start with a ten-hour window. I have been at it so long I love to go at least eighteen to twenty-four hours. Therefore, my eating window is typically four hours. However, I don't recommend beginning with a prolonged fast right away. It would be best if you worked up to that efficiency in the cells, which is why I created this program. Be patient and work your way up. As you get more fat adapted, you will burn more fat for energy, and you will be able to fast for longer periods. The idea is to do a short daily fast, only eating during certain hours of the day.

You decide your window time. Maybe you like to have breakfast in the morning. Perhaps you want to eat a later dinner. You pick your ten-hour window. You may think, "I can do better than that. I'm going to pick a six-hour window." My eating window is four to five hours every day. You might start with ten hours, and then decide you can move it to eight, then six, then four. You pick where you want to start and end, and you can always tweak it along the way.

How many meals do you consume during that window? You get to eat two meals in that window. The good news is you can take ninety minutes per meal, so take your time and consume adequate calories. Don't eat less; eat less often. If you do not consume enough calories during that window, eventually the body will think it's starving, and this lowers your metabolism and can make you gain weight. The key is eating less often and eating until you are full for at least one meal. My first meal is usually a quick midday meal because I am so busy, but at my dinner, I feast until full, so my body never feels like it's running out of fuel (starving).

If you don't consume enough calories, the body will want to conserve fat, and you will burn less of the fat for energy. This happened to me by going too low carb for a lengthy period. I was continuously lowering my carb intake, which worked initially. However, the fast loss stopped, and I gained belly fat. I dropped my carbs more (lower than 10 grams a day), and my body just held on to the fat. I realized I needed to throw in some higher carb meals to show my body it wasn't starving, and this has been my experience with multiple clients and for our doctors as well. We will dive further into diet variation in the next chapter, but for this week, focus on eating in the window and eating until you are full. You have ninety minutes or more if it's one meal.

An example is that you might stop all food intake after 7–8 pm, sleep, wake up the next morning, and except for non-sugary drinks, like pure water, organic coffee,[18] tea, you continue the fast until midday or even that evening. Consume food for that day between the hours of 2–8 pm. As you grow accustomed to intermittent fasting, you can push that window of time to be even more compressed.

Note: It's essential to stop eating three to four hours before bedtime, to not disrupt your deep recovery sleep.

You can choose your eating window. For example, let's say you have chosen to eat in an 8 hour window. You can have your first meal of the day at 12pm. Then your next meal could be at 7:00pm (your dinner), giving you an hour to eat before the window closes. You could also choose a shorter window like 2pm to 6pm for added benefits.

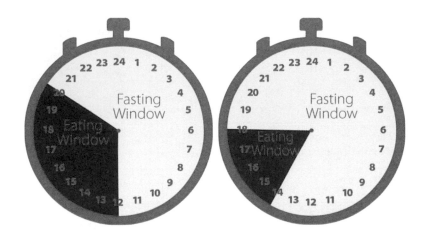

HOW CAN I DETERMINE MY BEST EATING WINDOW?

Your eating window is determined by the health of your mitochondria and your cells. It is always best to start with a smaller fasting window and a larger eating window. Over the years, I have developed a more exact way to determine your eating window. Your morning glucose and ketones, and your glucose and ketones before your first meal will help you figure this out. What we want to see is your glucose trending down, and your ketones trending up as you fast through the day. If this is not happening, then perhaps your fasting window is too large.

For example, if your morning glucose is 90, and ketones are .6 at 6 a.m. and then you test again before your first meal at noon and your glucose raises from 90 to 97 and your ketones lower from .6 to .5, these numbers would show that your mitochondria are not fat-adapting and are still using glucose as energy. It would show a need to shorten your fasting window by an hour or so and retest the next day. It is best to evaluate for three days to get a good average. Experiment with these numbers and find the best eating window for you. The numbers will correct over time with the strategies in this book. However, it's best to go slowly and start with a smaller fasting window. Periodically retest and reassess your window. The next step covered in the next chapter on diet variation is the solution for improved mitochondrial function and therefore, extending your fasting window. So please hang in there!

If you are not in ketosis by Week 3 (.5 or higher when measuring):

If	Then
If your morning blood ketone reading is not above .5	Reduce the number of carbs you are consuming. i.e. 10-20 grams for some people. To calculate your NET carbs per day: 1. For non-packaged food use an app such as Chronometer, which can tell you the correct amount of net carbs in various foods. 2. Formula: Total Daily Carbohydrates – Total Daily Fiber = NET Carbs Example: 150 carb – 90 fiber = 60 NET Carbs
Not losing weight or going into ketosis	• Drop down to LESS than 30 NET carbs per day. • Keep protein at one-half your body weight in grams. Example: 150-pound person should have 75 grams of protein a day.

Figure 3: Understand the relationship between NET carbs and achieving ketosis.

Take Note: Emotional stress increases cortisol, which increases glucose and decreases ketones, throwing your numbers off. Therefore, eliminate stressful days from your average. Exercise can also alter your numbers by reducing stored glucose. Therefore, do not test on exercise days.

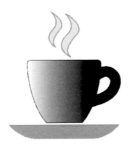

DOES COFFEE OR TEA IN THE MORNING RUIN MY FAST?

The answer to your question is this: I'm not sure; you need to test. Many of us love our coffee or tea in the morning. For some people, coffee or tea can spike glucose, and for some, it doesn't. If coffee or tea spikes glucose, then it will slow or stop your autophagy and is not suitable for you to drink during the fasting time. If coffee or tea does not raise glucose, then it's a go for you.

Remember the Keto-Mojo test I mentioned earlier? Check your glucose in the morning and recheck it thirty minutes after having your cup of coffee. You can also test it with and without fat in the coffee. Some get less rise or no rise from fat added, and some get more rise. In that case, try black coffee or try tea. If your glucose rises consistently above 5 or more each time you test after coffee with fat or without, you may be sensitive to coffee or caffeine and need to change to either tea or decaf. Then check those as well. If the number stays the same or drops, then coffee is not breaking you out of the autophagy state, and there will still be a rise in stem cells. Therefore, you should be fine to continue drinking coffee.

What about coffee?

Coffee affects everyone differently. Test your glucose first thing in the morning, have your coffee, and then test your glucose again 30 minutes later. If your glucose drops or stays the same, you can have coffee on this plan; if your glucose rises, you will have to forgo coffee throughout your Stemnomic journey. Different caffeine sources impact the body differently, so try separately for tea.

SAMPLE EATING WINDOW MEAL PLAN FOR WEEK 3

NOTE: Italicized items can be found in the *Meal Plans and Recipes* section.

Monday

Meal 1: (11 am) *Wild Blueberry Smoothie, Coconut Yogurt* with nuts and seeds

Meal 2: (6 pm) *Zucchini Noodles with Pesto and Beef Meatballs*

Tuesday

Meal 1: (11 am) *Purple Power Smoothie*

Meal 2: (6 pm) *Braised Beef Cheek Stew*

Wednesday

Meal 1: (11 am) Yogurt or kefir with fresh berries and nuts/seeds, drizzled with nut butter

Meal 2: (6 pm) *Braised Beef Cheek Stew* leftovers

Thursday

Meal 1: (11 am) Loaded Mexican-style *Omelet*, with shredded chicken, cheese, chives, parsley, coriander, salsa, and sour cream

Meal 2: (6 pm) Big green salad, with beef, tomatoes avocado, olive oil, and lemon juice

Friday

Meal 1: (11 am) *Probiotic Protein Powerhouse Smoothie*

Meal 2: (6 pm) Chicken Pad Thai with Shirataki noodles

Saturday

Meal 1: (11 am) Poached eggs on a bed of arugula, with grilled asparagus, avocado, and mushrooms

Meal 2: (6 pm) Grilled fish with cucumber, feta, tomato, and olive salad

Sunday

Meal 1: (11 am) Cucumber, tomato, feta, and olive salad with olive oil with lentils

Meal 2: (6 pm) *Zucchini Noodles with Pesto* and *Beef Meatballs*

DIET VARIATION FEAST/FAMINE CYCLING THE 5-1-1 RULE

Congratulations, you made it to Week 4! I like to refer to this week as *Feast/Famine Cycling*. You may not like the word famine, but the word feast has your attention, right? The principle behind this is utterly amazing.

Like most of what I teach, it comes from my own experiences. I was hardcore into ketosis when I noticed that I was gaining some odd belly fat, and I was losing strength and muscle, despite increasing my workout intensity. As many would do, I cut my carbs going from 50 grams of carbs/day down to within 30 grams, and then even below 10 grams. Things were getting worse, not better.

In my search for an answer, I found something that said long-term that low- carb dieting could cause insulin resistance. I thought to myself, "How can that be? Low-carb makes such a difference for diabetes?" However, what I found was that it wasn't insulin resistance like a person with diabetes, but an insulin resistance caused by the body's innate intelligence (inner wisdom to survive). Meaning, the cell turns down the receptor to insulin on the cell membrane, to blunt insulin's effect on the cell. Insulin is a fat-storing hormone, so this is a survival mechanism to hold on to the fat and store more. Why?

Simple! To survive. If fat is the body's main and only fuel, it will do everything it can to hold on to this precious fuel, at all costs, to survive. The point is, your metabolism slows, decreasing fat burning and energy. Oh, it gets worse! The body will break muscle down into glucose, using a process called gluconeogenesis. I was becoming "skinny fat" (trust me, not a good look).

Diet variation (feast/famine cycling) is how you rekindle and fire up the fat-burning machine. Recall from the earlier chapter; if you had to decrease your fasting window because of the glucose and ketone test, diet variation is the solution for broadening that window. Diet variation (feast/famine cycling) reminds the body it's not starving and to use fat as fuel at will.

From our growing group of Platinum practitioners trained in these strategies (Health Centers of the Future) and our Facebook fasting group, *Fasting for a Purpose*, we get much feedback from thousands of people from around the world, and we have learned what works. We also have learned what doesn't work.

When I discovered diet variation, it was an immediate breakthrough for so many struggling on low-carb diets or fasting. I'm telling you the results are extraordinary. For weight loss resistance and those with hormone conditions such as hypothyroid, adrenal fatigue, or hormone dysregulation, this will be a breakthrough for you. It's often said that women and those who have the previously stated conditions cannot do low-carb diets, ketosis, or fast, and that may be true if not using diet variation (feast/famine cycles). Variation works even for the healthy person trying to maximize their results in a low-carb diet, ketosis, fasting, or merely optimizing their hormones for health and longevity.

It's important to note that there are seasonal, monthly, and weekly variation strategies in this chapter proven effective by our group of trained

Platinum practitioners using the multi-therapeutic approach mentioned in the introduction.

You will see that these strategies go far beyond what to eat, where most diets focus, but rely on a far more important principle of adaptation (the body's drive to survive). My "feast/famine cycle" principle lies at the core and will change the way you look at diets, calories, hormones, and weight loss or weight gain forever.

REASONS TO VARY THE DIET

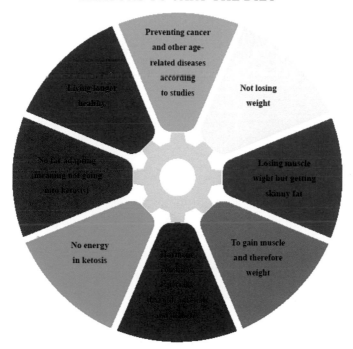

Preventing cancer and other age-related diseases according to studies

Not losing weight

Living longer healthy

No fat adapting (meaning not going into ketosis)

Losing muscle wight but getting skinny fat

No energy in ketosis

Hormone issues

To gain muscle and therefore weight

Most of us struggle with a few of these issues and hear it's all about eating more fat, less fat, fewer carbs, less protein, more protein, and for sure fewer calories. This information can be very confusing, and we struggle with choosing what to eat. When people get confused, they end up doing nothing.

WHICH DIET IS RIGHT?

There are new diets every time we turn around.

- The Paleo Diet
- The Ketogenic Diet
- Vegetarian Diets
- The Raw Food Diet
- The Super Carb Diet
- The T. Rex Diet (Carnivore Diet)—becoming popular right now.

KETO FOOD PYRAMID

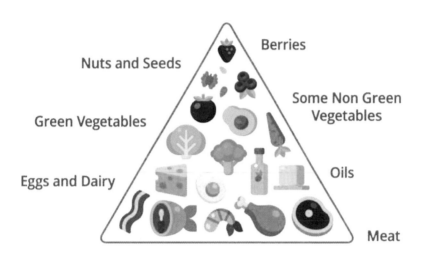

Nuts and Seeds

Berries

Green Vegetables

Some Non Green Vegetables

Eggs and Dairy

Oils

Meat

Exclude:

| Bread | Pasta | Sugar | Milk | Corn | Beans | Rice |

PALEO FOOD PYRAMID

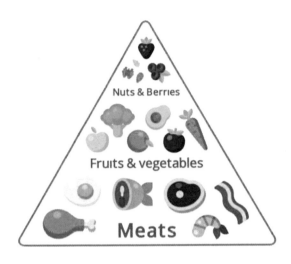

Nuts & Berries

Fruits & vegetables

Meats

Exclude:

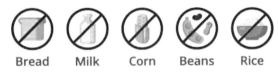

Bread   Milk   Corn   Beans   Rice

When speaking with die hard individuals in any of these camps above, we all hear how one specific diet changed their life, and how they will always eat this way from now on. These individuals will point to studies in favor of their diet, but most often, it is mainly their testimony to which they hold on. Who could blame them? After a person experiences positive results from a dietary change, the natural tendency is to remain on that diet. My first question is always: Did the results last? Meaning, are they still losing weight, or are they still feeling amazing?

With science, there are available published studies that support all these diets. So, which is right? Perhaps they all are. Here is the point: When you dig deeper into the scientific literature, the magic is not in the indefinite use of any one diet, but the dietary shift or change. When a person shifts from the standard American diet to a vegetarian or vegan diet, they feel better initially.

Similarly, going from any high-carbohydrate diet to a paleo diet will shift your health markers in a positive direction, and will give you consistent, lasting energy. However, like the best exercise routine, the results come in the beginning but fall off even to the point of feeling you are going backward. I have been collaborating with doctors and clients for many years and can tell you that, like exercise, staying in any one diet for too long almost always comes with negative consequences.

No healthy ancient culture stayed on any one diet continually as it was impossible. Environmental stressors from seasonal changes or harsh weather such as droughts and storms affected their diet. Even the lack of food or changes in food sources would force a dietary shift. Today we do not have these same stressors, and we have the option of staying on the same diet day in, day out because of continuous food availability which has led to some unique challenges and consequences of increased risk of several diseases and hormone problems.

The findings in the study, *Diet, Individual Responsiveness, and Cancer Prevention*, by M.J. Wargovich, make a strong point:

"The last half century has brought stark changes in lifestyle that depart from the normal diurnal cycle and periodic fluctuations in food availability. Thus, modern times are characterized as being constantly in a "feast" environment.

The cellular consequences may be an increase in risk for several diseases, including cancer."[1]

From both my clinical experience and digging deep into the contradictions in diet advice literature, I believe diet variation and feast/famine cycles are a unique answer that few are talking about and even less are using clinically. This one thing is the key to living longer healthy, and an answer for those with weight loss resistance, struggling on a low-carb diet, hormone conditions, and even cancer prevention. Diet variation (feast/famine cycles) is what our ancestors needed for survival and is programmed in our DNA.

New science presented in an article in the July 2018 issue of *Scientific American* shows our ancestors may not have eaten what we thought.[2] The old science looked at tooth shape, intestinal length, and other physical characteristics to determine what early humans ate. The new science, referred to as "footprints," looks at actual microbes and chew patterns in the teeth of the people themselves. This new method reveals a much more exact view of ancestral eating patterns, and it's not what we thought.

"This research revealed that our ancestors were very flexible eaters, who varied their diet based on changing climates, habitats, and food availability. The researchers believe this to be the key to their evolutionary success. Footprints teach us that early hominin diets varied over time and space, and we most likely evolved to be flexible eaters, driven by ever-changing climates."

THE SCIENCE

There are seasonal strategies, monthly strategies, and weekly strategies we can enforce. We will examine all of them as a part of this approach. All these strategies play a key role in something I refer to as *hormone optimization via adaptation*, which means we can optimize our hormones by forcing our bodies to adapt. The body's innate intelligence wants to survive at all costs.

If it feels threatened, to survive, it will marshal up an incredible surge of hormonal responses. Hormones release to increase heart rate to bring blood into our muscles and to become faster, stronger, and improve healing. Growth hormone and norepinephrine will drive this acute response but also provide us with a more lasting anti-aging, anti-inflammatory healing response.[3] Even our cells become more sensitive to our hormones which are the key to feeling amazing,[4] living longer healthy, and an answer to most hormone-related conditions like thyroid, diabetes, obesity, and weight loss resistance.[5]

Many people know the benefits of growth hormones. However, norepinephrine, also called noradrenaline, is less appreciated.[6] Norepinephrine acts to increase the force of skeletal muscle contraction, and the rate and force of contraction of the heart in acute stress to save our life.[7] The actions of norepinephrine are vital to the flight or fight response, whereby the body prepares to react to or retreat from an acute threat.

We enjoy long-term effects as well because it also acts to decrease inflammation, especially in the brain.[8] Norepinephrine also brings balance to other brain neurotransmitters—chemicals the brain has, which are essential for function. It is a part of most neurodegenerative and brain conditions such as Parkinson's, Alzheimer's, ADHD, bipolar disorder, anxiety, mood disorders, and depression.[9] Studies showing lower levels of norepinephrine somehow connect to all these conditions. Studies also show that periodic surges play a significant role in prevention and possible treatment of these conditions.[10]

Many drugs are being developed around both important anti-aging hormones. However, it is my opinion that merely forcing the body to adapt is still the only safe and predictable way to perfect these incredible hormones, without negatively affecting other systems. We can do this through dietary changes weekly, monthly, and seasonally. To fully understand how this works, I will present some typical strategies the use of which you may be familiar, including cold therapy (cryotherapy), hyper and hypo oxygen, and exercise.

Less typical, yet I believe to be more powerful, are diet shifts and feast/ famine cycles. Let's start with exercise because it is perhaps the easiest example in understanding the principles behind diet variation.

When you begin an exercise program, you typically get immediate results. The body adapting to the stress of the exercise drives the results. Exercise, like dietary shifts, will raise growth hormone-making cells more sensitive to your other hormones such as insulin and increasing norepinephrine. Like diet, if you continue to do the same exercise day in, day out, there is no need for the body to adapt, because the adaptation occurred. Therefore, the results typically level off. The moment you force adaptation through changing your routine, the results start up again.

Bodybuilders figured this out years ago. It's not the next miracle device or program in the marketplace; it's the exercise variation or change that makes the most difference. Infomercials make money because most people don't understand this principle. We think it's the next new thing—P90X, TRX, or Ab Blaster—that we must have to be fit and lose weight. Truthfully, it's not the diet or the next exercise program we need; it is the hormone optimization driven by the adaptation.

Another notable example of this (one which I experienced) is cryotherapy. I interviewed a gentleman on *Cellular Healing TV* from C1 Recovery Cryotherapy. According to him, everyone struggles with inflammation. Cryotherapy flushes this inflammation from the body. The principle of cryotherapy is like that of diet variation. The rise in growth hormone and norepinephrine that occurs is why it works. Studies show that cryotherapy stimulates the burning of fat, reduces inflammation, and creates a general feeling of well-being.[11] It is impressive how well it works.

The same principle applies to long and short-term stress meaning that short-term stress and adaptation are good and create all the positive benefits mentioned, but long-term stress can contribute to inflammation and disease. A good example is cryotherapy—the short-term stress is three minutes, and the body adapts, and all is amazing. However, stay in six minutes, and you're dead. Too much of any stress, whether it's emotional or physical exercise, could be bad if the body does not adapt. As you can see, the key here is the adaptation via hormone optimization.

There was a study done with mice, moving them in and out of cold temperatures forcing adaptation, which resulted in dramatic weight loss. In the study, they found that part of the adaptation was the gut bacteria known as the *microbiome*. Many studies have shown that our gut microbiome plays a vital role in our metabolism, and therefore, in most aspects of our healthy weight loss or gain. In this study, they noted a specific microbe associated with obesity and diabetes virtually disappeared when exposed to cold temperatures. The shift in the microbiome was part of the adaptation to survive; however, it led to a hormone optimization and therefore weight loss.[12]

There are theories that seasonal dietary changes cause similar shifts or adaptation of the microbiome and are part of why we see such positive results with hormone conditions and gut healing. I can speak from a clinical perspective that we see incredible results with the most challenging gut cases using diet variation seasonally and monthly and weekly as explained below. Some believe that our microbiome shifts seasonally based on the sun's position or perhaps other factors, but it is the shift in the microbiome that sets up the need to change our diets. Either way, we know the bacteria in our gut are part of this need for diet changes and part of why it works.

Ancient cultures unknowingly benefited survival and their long-term health by being forced into times of diet changes and feast/famine cycles. Many studies show that growth hormone and norepinephrine increase during fasting states as part of the adaptation for survival.[13]

The rise in the hormones and the increase in hormone sensitivity drives fat adaptation and the preservation of lean muscle mass. One study shows that the norepinephrine release from abrupt diet shifts (alternate day fasting) was the key to more significant weight loss. The study compared a high-fat diet, low-fat diet, low-carb and high-carb diet eaten daily, meaning seven days a week, and not alternated with a fast day. Then each diet was eaten every other day, alternating with a fast day. For example, they ate one day of high-fat or low-carb food throughout the day, then the next day, a fast day consisting of just one meal of high fat. The following day was another day of regular eating of the high-fat or low- carb meals. This alternate day fasting was also done with the low-fat diet.

The alternate day fasting worked better than the daily high-fat diet alone and the daily low-fat diet. This research showed that feast/famine produced a higher rise in norepinephrine. The hormone optimization (rise in norepinephrine) driven by the forced adaptation increased the lean muscle and caused a more significant loss of body fat.[14]

The diet variation was more important than the diet itself—this result held for the low-fat diet and the high-fat diet. Once again, perhaps all the diets are correct, but it's the variation that matters most.

The science is all around this principle, yet so few are teaching this. This study shows that intermittent energy restriction was superior to continued energy restriction. So, the research shows that intermittent caloric restriction is better for weight loss, metabolic diseases, and anti-aging than constant caloric restriction.[15]

This study will convince you it is less about the food and more about the hormone optimization created by the adaptation of diet change (feast/ famine). One group ate a diet of 25–30% restricted calories in three meals a day every day, compared to another group eating five days a week whatever they wanted and the other two days a week at 500 calories (5-2 diet). It is important to note that the weekly caloric intake was the same for both groups, so the results were not based on calories. Here is a quote from the author Dr. Mark Mattson, Chief of the Laboratory of Neurosciences at the National Institute on Aging and Professor of Neuroscience at Johns Hopkins University:

"We saw superior beneficial effects of 5–2 diet on glucose regulation (a risk factor for diabetes) and loss of belly fat (a risk factor for cardiovascular disease) compared to the women eating regular meals but restricting calories."

It utterly amazes me that more people are not teaching and implementing this type of variation. The science is one thing, but as a group of doctors using these strategies clinically, it is a real breakthrough for so many people struggling, even for those like my wife and myself who want to take their health to the next level. It has been a blessing to us in so many ways, especially being in our 50s. If this were not enough, the hormone optimization gets better.

RAISE YOUR TESTOSTERONE NATURALLY

It's worth noting that the rise in a hormone known as luteinizing hormone, the precursor for testosterone (T), is significant during a fasting state which also accounts for some fantastic results we see with even short daily fasts. This study showed a short-term fast increased luteinizing hormone by a staggering 67% in non-obese males. Obese males showed a 26% increase.

There was a 180% increase in T in the non-obese group.[16]

"All this hormone optimization is great, but the fact is, I am still struggling."

As said before, some people in the health community believe that people with hormone issues, thyroid conditions, and adrenal fatigue are not candidates for low-carb diets, ketosis, or fasting. It's also often thought that women, should not follow a low-carb diet, ketosis, or a fast. The common complaints are low energy, generally feeling "horrible," thinning brittle hair, inability to lose weight, and worse yet, fat gain. These complaints are a reality for many; however, diet variation (feast/famine cycle) is the answer, even for those who struggle to get into ketosis.

My wife's experience is classic for so many and illustrates this point well. She was never overweight. However, she struggled to fat adapt in ketosis. The mitochondria in her cells were not working well. Like most people living in today's environment, she was stuck as a sugar burner not hormonally efficient at using fat for energy. You may say, "Why was she not fat?" Most thin people, who are sugar burners, store fat in their organs, and this can be worse for their health than when you store fat on your body. Her breakthrough and the fat burning transition was through diet variation.

MY WIFE MERILY'S EXPERIENCE

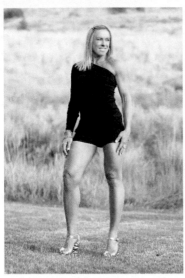

"My wife more fit in her 50s than when I met her at age

My first attempt at getting into ketosis was a fail. I even dropped my carb intake to less than 10 grams a day for a week or so. That was difficult, but I was willing to do whatever it took to adapt. When that didn't work, my husband suggested resuming my typical diet (grain free/sugar- free as was typical with infrequent and only ancient grains). This diet was higher in healthy carbs, most likely averaging 200 grams/day. After a month, I tried getting into ketosis again, and according to the numbers on the meter, I was in ketosis after a week, but barely.

After a few months, I went back to the higher, healthier carbohydrate diet once again, and even became a bit less committed to eating as strictly as usual. I then went back into ketosis again, and even added in a few feast days of eating whatever, including breakfast. These were not as fun as they sound since I would become more tired earlier. It wasn't until I fasted a few times that I found my responsiveness to the process becoming more efficient, and fat adaptation became less challenging.

Our culture of "quick fixes" is unrealistic in value. I see through the artful deception of expecting the process in many areas of life development to be without cost or pain, which is not only improbable but impossible.

Since this time, Daniel has been applying those "tricks" that he "pulled" on me with others, and it is repeatedly proving itself to work. The lesson is not to get frustrated, but to use what you learn here, which works, and stay the course, and eventually, the body responds like magic. Many want a "quick fix" to their challenges. That is never the case with what truly works, but following the principles he teaches does work, though it often takes a while to arrive at the destination. The learning that occurs in all journeys in life is, in fact, the destination. So why would this be any different?

THE SIMPLE ANSWER FOR WHY YOU ARE
NOT FAT-ADAPTING OR LOSING WEIGHT

As seen in my own story of long-term low-carb or low-calorie diet, the body will try to preserve its precious fuel supply two ways to which you can relate:

1. The body will slow lipolysis (fat-burning) by taking up more water in the fat cell and producing fat deposits called cellulite.[17]

2. The body will blunt insulin receptors to hold on to its precious fat.[18] Insulin is a fat-storing hormone, and if the body blunts the cell receptors to it, you will hold more fat.[19] This process is great for survival but bad for your belly or thighs. We often hear that ketosis or low-carb diets cause insulin resistance like Type 2 diabetes, which is driven by disease. However, it is different because the body can reverse the insulin resistance very quickly once it feels there is no need to hold on to its fat for survival. Disease does not drive this type of insulin resistance, only an adaptation to survive.

What if you live deep in Alaska in the heart of winter and have only one source of fuel like a big wood pile (your fat, the state of ketosis, or low- carb diet, in this example), and the winter is getting colder and longer. Will you burn more wood or less as the hard winter goes on as you see the pile dwindling quickly? If you want to survive, you will burn less and less and be happy at say 60 degrees instead of 75 degrees. Your body is no different with its precious fuel of fat. If this is its only fuel, it will find ways to burn less with one goal only—survival.

Now let's say that an old friend stops by to check up on you during the hard winter. He notices you have little wood left and offered you some of his wood because he has plenty. Will you now burn more or less? You will start to burn more and bring your home back up to a warm 75 degrees again. No different from if we offer our body a feast day, it will fire up the fat-burning again, and two days later you will see higher ketone numbers as a sign of more fat-burning and a visible difference in how you look. **Weekly diet variation with its feast/famine cycles is the simple answer.**

WEEKLY DIET VARIATION, FEAST AND FAMINE 5-1-1 RULE

Adding in even one feast day a week to remind the body it's not starving is magic. The 5-1-1 is a weekly diet variation strategy and does just that.

The 5-1-1 looks like this:

One "feast day" sets up variation and reminds the body it's not starving. It also stimulates a pathway known as mTOR.[20] This pathway stimulates a hormone called Igf1 that causes cell growth and a very anabolic effect.

Bodybuilders love this pathway and use strategies to stimulate the pathway to increase muscle growth. They increase and force calories, carbs, and protein.[21] It is a feast far beyond one or two days. The problem is that studies show that staying long term in this pathway has links to cancer, diabetes, and aging.[22] However, short times in this pathway can be healing. In a growth phase, the body can heal very quickly but stay in that pathway like a long-term paleo high-protein diet, and you can end up with health issues. When bodybuilders first enter this phase, they boast of how good their joints feel and their energy is amazing. However, it is short-lived, and later, unknowingly leads to health problems.

The opposite side of the coin is autophagy, one of my favorite pathways as you know by now. The three diet changes that stimulate this action are a decrease in calories, carbs, and protein,[23] the exact opposite of mTOR. I will argue that too much time in this pathway is not good either. There is a negative effect on the immune system, along with organ and muscle wasting. You will find this with vegetarians or vegans.

Feast Famine Drives Major Adaptation and Hormone Optimization

mTor: Cell Replicating & Anabolic

1. Feasting (days/weeks)
2. Increased calories (days/weeks)
3. High Carb (100-200g a day)

4. High Protein (100-200g a day)

Autophagy: Cell Cleaning and Catabolic

1. Fasting (daily or extended)
2. Restricted calories (partial fast or a fasting mimicking diet)
3. Low carb (keto)
4. Low protein (under 20g a day)

I repeat: The magic lies in both feast and famine. Short term in both brings healing, and it is the variation that creates the adaptation that drives the hormone optimization and the changes to the microbiome that lead to the results we see clinically and in studies. I argue we need both the 5-1-1 and the 4-2-1, as well as the monthly variation that we will discuss next.

The 5-1-1 strategy is one feast day and one famine day. The famine day (fast day) will drive autophagy, growth hormone, and hormone sensitivity. The longer fast days, compared to the daily fast on the five days of intermittent fasting, challenges the mitochondria where you burn fat and produce energy to adapt. Cells with defective mitochondria do not adapt and die. This process is the basis for my Metabolic Mitochondrial Fitness (MMF) concept. Like exercise, if you push it, it will either adapt and get stronger with better function and fat-burning abilities or die. Either way, you win because you will raise stem cells after the autophagy and make better, stronger cells with better mitochondria. This fact is the basic principle behind *Beyond Fasting*.

The 5-1-1 strategy forces more adaptation to optimize hormones to become more efficient fat burners. The more fat adapted you are by the time of the fast, the more autophagy and stem cells you produce and therefore, the greater your results.

The 5-1-1 strategy will also be the answer for those who struggle metabolically with low-carb diets, fasting, or intermittent fasting and those with thyroid and adrenal issues. I find the benefit is more significant for women, and many of you will benefit even more by adding in the monthly diet variation strategy.

MONTHLY DIET VARIATION

There is another answer to why you are not fat-adapting or feeling well. Five to seven days of a feast could change your hormones for the rest of the month.

High healthy carbs associated with a feast day will drive up insulin levels through the mTOR pathway. Long-term elevated insulin has many noticeable adverse effects like obesity, cancer, diabetes, and aging. However, a short term can transform your hormones by helping to convert inactive hormones to active hormones.

Insulin carries many roles in its relation to other hormones, especially about the hormone convergence. Hormone convergence means hormones need to convert from one form to another for active use. One of the best examples of this conversion is thyroid hormone. Thyroid hormone T3 is the active form of the hormone that helps our body (cells) use fat for energy. Active Free T3 has many other functions, such as overall health of our skin and hair, and even daily energy. Therefore, if your cells don't get enough or its message, you will not feel well or burn fat normally or efficiently. T4 is the inactive form that must convert to the active T3. The lack of converting T3 will affect how you feel and use fat for energy. We need insulin for this conversion to take place.

Therefore, if insulin is low for too long, the lack of active T3 can become a problem. Those on a low-carb diet for extended periods can develop deficient insulin that will affect not only fat loss and muscle loss but also other hormones. People who already have hormone challenges are even more sensitive to this potential problem and respond the best to what I refer to as monthly diet variation.

One healthy high-carb week a month, or at least five days as described below, pushes up the insulin and not only helps the conversion of T4 to T3 but other hormones like estrogen and testosterone. The week before a woman's period is when we have discovered the best time to drive the insulin up to aid in the many hormonal needs that take place. Think about how smart the body is. Most women would say this is when they get the cravings for carbs and sugar.

Listen to your body, but reach for the healthy carbs like fruits, sweet potatoes, yams, ancient grains, ground vegetables, and so forth.

This strategy is a proven one for men, as well. The variation strategy reminds your body it has plenty and is not starving, and the variation of the increased carbs or protein drives the mTOR pathway, which again is an anabolic pathway for growth and healing if used short term. Short-term stimulation of this pathway from high carbs, protein, or calories can have a healing effect and even improve the hormones and metabolism. I do agree to look at the studies which show that long-term in this state can have detrimental negative effects.

Many ask me how long to stay on a high protein or carb diet safely. I can only say that what I saw in Africa was feast/famine. When they had a kill, they were in high protein for days to a week. When they didn't, they could be high carb if they had that or a famine or a drought. The Hunza people, one of the longest living, healthiest ancient cultures on the planet, have a diet where summer food is plant-based, autumn is high carb with more fruits and root vegetables, and they are completely in ketosis in the winter. By spring, they go into a fasting state which they refer to as "Fasting Spring" because it became such an important part of their culture. It is the consistent yearly fast that is the key to their longevity and health. The point is that they were forced into diet variation and feast/famine cycles, which led to their health and longevity. I believe our DNA is set up for this adaptation. However, since today, we are not forced into this adaptation, we must plan it.

Either one week or short sessions of high-protein or high-carb emulating a feast state can be a game changer for most. I believe it is even needed to create the adaptation and therefore, hormone optimization most people need today to feel well. A way to emulate the Hunza tribe using a monthly variation is to do five days a month of high healthy carbs or high protein and choose another random five days to water fast or partial fast or do a fasting mimicking diet. My doctors and I use this strategy for many of our patients and clients who struggle hormonally or need to break through weight loss resistance.

ARE YOU LOSING MUSCLE AND GAINING FAT ON A LOW-CARB DIET?

Diet variation is also an answer for those who are losing muscle following a low-carb or ketogenic diet. I wrote about this concept in Chapter 10 of Dr. Joseph Mercola's book, *Fat for Fuel*, a great read, and resource.

Dr. Mercola was in ketosis for some time and was asking me about muscle loss. I explained to him our success with adding in feast days. This strategy was the answer for him as it had been for me. Dr. Mercola was grateful and asked me to write a section in his book explaining how we need to remind the body it is not starving and of the need to keep fat-burning active by using high protein or high carb days weekly.

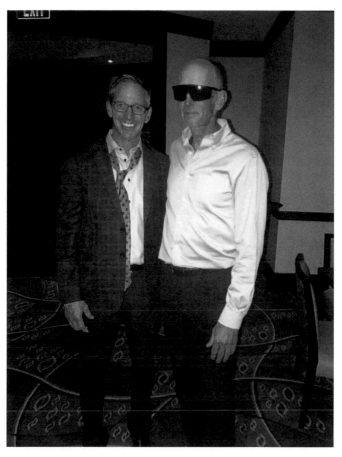

One of insulin's functions is turning off gluconeogenesis, which is making glucose from a non-carbohydrate source such as glycerol or protein a from muscle.[24] Chronically low insulin, frequent in more extended periods of low-carb diets, can allow the body to use muscle as a preferred fuel source. So, as insulin drops, glucose can start to rise via gluconeogenesis.

There are many theories around why this affects some more than others, but some people are more prone to this. Understand that the body's innate ability to adapt and survive rules, so it is trying to help you survive. In other words, the body wants to hold on to its energy stores (stored fat or glucose stored as glycogen in the liver), so it will slowly use muscle and turn it into glucose for energy via gluconeo-genesis.[25] Another option is to dump glucose from the liver; however, one theory suggests that it wants to hold on to emergency fuel that is fast and easy to use just in case it must run from a predator. The body will go for muscle to break down into sugar before it uses its precious stored glucose.

Gluconeogenesis is hormone-driven for survival to keep energy stable. When energy is needed, and insulin is low from inadequate carb intake for prolonged periods, the body keeps its fat because that's what it is now using as a major energy source. As stated the body will also desire to keep the stored glucose (called glycogen) in the liver and muscles in case it needs fast energy to run and save its life.[26] The stored glucose is the fastest form of energy, so it makes sense it is smart enough to hold on to it.[27]

There are many hormones involved here, and studies show that insulin plays a leading role. This study shows in healthy individuals, insulin suppresses gluconeogenesis by 20%, while glycogenolysis (glucose made from stored glucose called glycogen) completely suppresses.[28] The study also points out[29] that insulin controls gluconeogenesis not just in the liver but also other tissues such as muscle.[30]

All the body wants to do is survive. Survival is its priority, at the cost of our concern to stay lean and hold muscle. Therefore, it will go for the muscle and keep the belly fat. Unfortunately, over time, the body gets more efficient at using muscle, so as we age, we tend to get "skinny fat." Not a great look. I can tell you personally because when I was sick, my body loved to use my muscle as fuel. People will even find that when they eat carbs, at times, their glucose will drop. The rise in insulin pulls the glucose in the cell and slows gluconeogenesis, especially in the liver.

More importantly, if they continue to use high carb days periodically, they will start to spare their muscle and will eventually start burning fat again. The increase in carbs will stop the gluconeogenesis and lower the glucose. This action can also cause a reverse effect. Continuing carbs day in, day out can give the body too much fuel, and it will start storing it again for another day. We gain body fat and store fat in our organs.

As you can see, it's not so black and white. This built-in hormonal survival mechanism complicates what we think should happen, or even expect to happen. The bottom line is that we can bio-hack this survival mechanism through intermittently reminding the body it has plenty of food to survive. We do so by either increasing calories, protein, or carbohydrates. The key word here is intermittent. Carbohydrates seem to work the most efficiently; however, we have found that some people react better to higher calorie or protein days.

BEYOND THE SCIENCE: MY OWN AFRICAN EXPERIENCE

My African experience was the changing factor in eating less often (intermittent fasting). However, it was also the first time I experienced feast/famine cycling firsthand. There are times when food is plenty, and times of drought where little food is available. They told me that the times of drought could be frequent, which would require longer periods of fasting.

The tribe I visited had recently come out of the mountainous area because of a prolonged drought. Many other tribes in this area received relief foods during the droughts. With these processed foods came modern diseases. This tribe did not take the food, as they were holding to their traditions and normal ways of hunting and gathering.

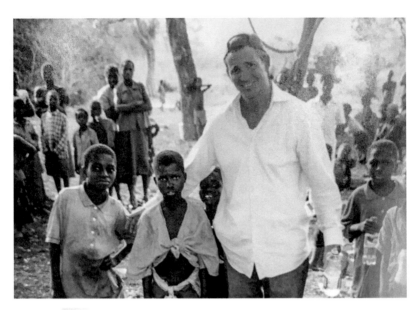

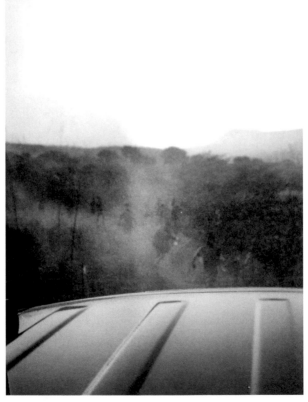

One question asked by the men who brought me was, "Why don't they have diseases like the other tribes?" Not only did they have no disease to speak of, but their level of fitness, even the children, was extraordinary. The children chased us in and out of the bush for miles and miles. Their conditioning stunned us. One guide explained that there are times of little food because of droughts, mentioning how the tribal diets varied significantly based on the seasons and what was available. People foraged wild plants when they could and sacrificed a goat when no other meat was available.

This concept of feast and famine is how we have adapted for survival. Eating in correspondence with the seasons was the first thing our ancestors did correctly, not that they had a choice. Also, our ancestors did not sit down for three square meals and several snacks throughout the day. The ever-changing environment required them to follow a feast or famine style of life characterized by alternating periods when food was either in abundance or short supply. Contrary to widespread belief, those periods of lack and abundance of food were beneficial to their health

The body is designed to survive. Our DNA is programmed for it as part of our innate survival mechanism. Times of famine turn on specific genes that decrease inflammation, prevent disease, and even promote longer and healthier life, and recent studies are teaching us that these fasting states are key for health and longevity. We are more prone to disease without them.

WEEKLY DIET VARIATION 5-1-1: FEAST AND FAMINE "HOW TO"

The 5-1-1 feast and famine cycling includes five days of regular intermittent fasting; one day of complete fast or one day with a meal (in 24 hours) or a partial fast (the famine day); and one day of increased carbohydrate/protein and general calories day (the feast day).

The Famine (Fast) Day

We're challenging the mitochondria to tap into those fat stores.[31] We're getting the mitochondria to use fat as an energy source. We're also getting more autophagy. Studies show that after fifteen hours of fasting, the body destroys more of the bad cells, and increases stem cell production.[32] Once we get past the fifteen-hour mark, these changes begin to take place. For the fast day, you may want to fast all day but start by just picking one meal. So maybe that's 6:00 at night, and you have dinner. That's your meal. Maybe you choose an earlier time, such as 3:00. The point is, make it simple. Just choose one meal and eat it. That's your fasting day. You can also eat just 500-800 calories and keep protein under 15-20 grams in that meal instead of a full meal. We call this a partial fast. The limited calories and protein for a brief time stimulates autophagy just like a pure water fast (more on partial fasting later) but is easier than a full day without food.

The Feast Day

Here's the fun part, the feast day. Pick one day where you purposely eat more, and even up your carbohydrate intake. I typically feast on a weekend, and I up my carbohydrates from vegetable sources, fruits, potatoes, sweet potatoes, or yams. Sometimes I add more ancient grains like rice, quinoa, barley, Kamut, oats, spelt, and even wheat (I'm not gluten sensitive like I was when I was sick). Don't add grains if you don't do well with them. I try to get my carbs up to around 100 grams that day and up to 200. Why? We want to remind the body it isn't starving.

We added a famine day and added the feast day. Can you do them back to back? Yes, however, I like to separate them. I don't typically plan my famine days. I make them my busy days, and it can be any day during the week. I love doing my feast days on the weekend where I can enjoy a variety of healthy food with my family. I'm telling you; it is essential to keeping you on the plan. It allows you to fire up the fat-burning machine! It is that simple, five days of eating window, one feast, one famine.

REMINDER: By now you understand that caloric restriction doesn't work long-term. Even on your five intermittent fasting days, eating one meal completely to full, will tell your body you are not starving. One to two days a week or five days a month is fine for your fasting days, but continual caloric restriction will lead to problems. If you eat fewer calories, push food aside (like most of America does), your body will eventually think it's starving, lower the metabolism to survive, and hold on to fat. Don't eat less, eat less often! Even when you do eat less often, eat one meal until full. The important message is to tell your body it's not starving.

5-1-1-Rule

- For five days of the week, eat a ketogenic diet, and check your blood ketones to make sure you're in ketosis.

- During those five days, be sure to get the 2-2-2-2.

- One day of the week is a fasting day to support detoxification and give your digestive system a rest.33 Fasting has many proven benefits,34, but most importantly, it down-regulates inflammation, which helps to heal almost any health concern. You can choose to:

  1. Fast only on water for twenty-four hours and even into the next day.

  2. Do a partial fast (consuming 500-800 calories and protein under 15-20 grams) where you restrict food intake to a certain time window in the day (i.e. 1 pm -7 pm while skipping breakfast, or in one meal). Fasting accelerates fat-burning, but only once you are fat adapted. Once adapted, your body burns fat during a fasting state; however, if you're not adapted and fasting, your body may burn more muscle than fat.

- One day of the week is a fun "carb-load" or "protein-load" day. The carb-load day serves to refill your glycogen stores and reminds your body that it is not starving. The protein-load day seems to work better for some of our clients and patients, especially those who are carb sensitive. You can alter load days every other week (one-week carb load, the following week protein load, and so forth), depending on what works best for your body, health goals, and condition.

5-1-1 Weekly Example

FIVE days of regular intermittent fasting/ keto. Eat a ketogenic diet and check your blood ketones to make sure you're in ketosis. During these 5 days, follow the 2-2-2-2 rule:

- Add 2 Tbs. MCT or coconut oil
- Add 2 Tbs. high quality salt
- Add 2 Tbs. grass-fed organic butter
- Add 2 Tbs. olive oil
- Intermittent fast 15-18 hours

ONE day of complete or partial fasting (the famine day). Choose:

- Water fast all day
- One meal a day (eat to satiety). 22-24 hour dinner-to-dinner or breakfast-to-breakfast fasts.
- Partial fasting: 500-800 calories and under 20 grams of protein.
- Eat in small window, around 6 hours.

ONE day of increased carbohydrate OR increased protein (the feast day). Eat up to 100-200 grams of healthy carbs OR protein). The carb (or protein) load day serves to refill your glycogen stores, and reminds your body that it is not starving.

- Pick one day where you (with intention) eat more. Focus on increasing your carbohydrate (OR protein) intake particularly.
- Choose carbohydrates from nutrient-dense sources like sweet potatoes, yams, fruit, or ancient grains. Carbs (or protein) up to around 100-200 grams to remind the body that it isn't starving.

Example 5/1/1 week:

Monday	Tuesday	Wednesday	Thursday	Friday	Saturday	Sunday
Eating Window	Eating Window	Famine Day	Eating Window	Eating Window	Feast Day	Eating Window

Now choose your week:

Monday	Tuesday	Wednesday	Thursday	Friday	Saturday	Sunday

Figure 9: Remove the daily guess-work by using this chart to pre-select your diet variation days.

SAMPLE 5-1-1 FEAST/FAMINE CYCLING MEAL PLAN

NOTE: Italicized items can be found in the *Meal Plans and Recipes* section.

Monday

Meal 1 (Noon): *Chocolate Avocado Pudding, Homemade Coconut Yogurt* with nuts, seeds

Meal 2 (6 pm): *Cauliflower Crust Pizza* topped with pesto, chicken, and arugula

Tuesday

Meal 1 (Noon): Poached eggs on a bed of arugula, with grilled asparagus, avocado, and mushrooms

Meal 2 (6 pm): *Roasted Leg of Lamb with Mint Yogurt* and *Garlic Green Beans*

Wednesday

(FAMINE DAY: 1 meal, or fast all together)

Meal 1 (4 pm): *Green Soup* with avocado, toasted seeds, drizzled with olive oil

Thursday

    Meal 1 (Noon): *Probiotic Protein Powerhouse Smoothie*

    Meal 2 (6 pm): Chicken Pad Thai with shirataki noodles

Friday

    Meal 1 (Noon): *Omelet*, with grilled asparagus, prosciutto, and cheese

    Meal 2 (6 pm): Grilled fish with cucumber, feta, tomato, and olive salad

Saturday

    Meal 1 (Noon): *Chocolate Avocado Pudding*

    Meal 2 (6 pm): *Zucchini Noodles with Pesto and Beef Meatballs*

Sunday: Feast Day

    Meal 1 (Noon): *Omelet* with feta, vegetables, and avocado, and a sweet potato muffin with lots of butter and cinnamon

    Meal 2 (6 pm): Crispy salmon pan fried in ghee, with charred asparagus and oven roasted beetroot "chips"

DIET VARIATION FEAST/FAMINE CYCLING, THE 4-2-1 RULE

L ast week we focused on 5-1-1 feast/famine cycling. This week we will take it to the next level of feast/famine cycling, the 4-2-1 cycle. Are you ready to bring your fat-burning and autophagy to the next level? All you need to do this week is to add another fast day. This addition emulates the ancient cultures we discussed previously, challenging your mitochondria more, and preparing your body to fast. As said in the last chapter, the science fully supports feast/famine cycling, and we are just bringing it one step further.[1]

As we add on fasting days, it increases the Metabolic Mitochondrial Fitness (MMF). Through creating mitochondrial stress from increased fasting days, the cells must adapt. Bad cells do not adapt. Therefore, your body (via autophagy and stem cells) will get rid of the bad and create the new. This process is the basis for the *Stemnomic Principle*, a phrase you most likely have not heard because the science is so new about this topic, I had to create a word to reference it. Therefore, here is the proper definition: The Stemnomic Principle is the use of therapeutic strategies that enhance the production of stem cells. Here, we are using dietary strategies to create a stress on the cells that drives a process of cellular recycling (autophagy) and cellular renewal (stem cell activation), I spoke about in the introduction.

After a period, you end up with more efficient cells and mitochondria, with a greater ability to produce energy from fat, and therefore go longer periods without food. As a result, you are relying on your fat stores (fat adapted). Like exercise, the more you stress the muscle, the more efficient it becomes, the stronger you get, and the better you feel.[2]

HOW DO WE BREAK UP THIS WEEK?

I prefer to separate the two fasting days, so they are not back to back. For example, fast on Monday (either eating one meal or going all day without consuming food), then on Tuesday and Wednesday you intermittent fast within the window upon which you have decided. Then on Thursday, you fast again; Friday you intermittent fast; and on Saturday, you feast. This schedule is just an example, and you can mix it up in any way that feels best for you.

WHY ARE WE BRINGING THIS CYCLING TO THE NEXT LEVEL THIS WEEK?

We want to prepare your body for next week, where you undertake (possibly your first?) five-day fast. At this point, I genuinely believe you are ready for it. You have given your body adequate time to adjust to eating less by eating less often, increasing fat intake, and decreasing processed carbohydrates. This five-day fast coming up next week will bring about seven amazing accomplishments towards healing, which we will break down for you in the next chapter. This process is exciting!

This next step is especially important to get the most out of this program. We are creating more mitochondrial stress by increasing feast and famine. The more pressure we put on the cells, the more adaptation, and therefore, the more hormone optimization, fat adaptation, autophagy, and stem cell production. To go back and forth from the fast days (autophagy pathway that is used for recycling) and feast days (mTOR pathway used for regeneration) is the key to why this works.

MORE STRESS =

MORE ADAPTATION =

MORE HORMONE OPTIMIZATION =

MORE FAT ADAPTATION =

MORE AUTOPHAGY =

MORE STEM CELL PRODUCTION

Let's discuss the feast day of this week. The feast day doesn't have to be a higher carb day if you are not feeling it. Some people find that going higher protein on their feast days feels better. The important thing is that you are increasing your calories, protein, or carbs on feast days in a way that feels best to you. Any of the three will stimulate the building pathway mTOR, which is part of why this works. The results of the feast day are threefold: It's rewarding to let go and enjoy partaking in different foods (which is why I like to do so on a weekend day), and it also helps you to burn more fat rather than holding onto fat. It's reminding your body you are not starving, which is a vital part of feast/famine cycling.

Finally, the high carb or protein also stimulates the mTOR pathway that is a building and cell- replicating pathway. If you recall, this is the pathway that bodybuilders love because they put on muscle. However, recall that studies show that staying in this pathway too long leads to premature aging and disease from cell growth. On the short term, it can drive healing from the anabolic cell-replicating effect. Therefore, one to two days a week or five days a month harness the replenishing, repair, and renewal we achieve from the growth pathway. Some people do well with two feast days a week, which would be called a 3-2-2. Now you have two feast days and two fast days. We find this to be the case for thyroid and adrenal people.

When ancient cultures had food, they feasted. As I stated before, I watched the tribe I spent time with eating high amounts of protein, but it was only for a few days before going back to very little when finishing the catch.

Now the fast days. By adding a day of fasting, we increase the pressure on the cells to adapt, gaining more hormone optimization needed for the adaptation and more autophagy.

What this means for you is more fat-burning ability, metabolic flexibility (meaning you can move in and out of fat-burning amazingly fast), and more consistent energy. We call this mitochondrial fitness because this is where you teach your cells to burn fat, and at one week before the fast, it's time to fire up your fat-burning engines.

4-2-1 RULES

- For four days of the week, eat within an eating window. Maybe it's a four-hour window; maybe it's a six-hour window. Maybe you started at a ten-hour window but have made your way down to six hours. Just try to progress. I would try to shrink the eating window to create more mitochondrial stress. Test, as discussed in Chapter 3.

- During those four days of intermittent fasting, you are eating (two) meals within that eating window you chose.

- During those four days of intermittent fasting, be sure to stay on a ketogenic diet, keeping carbohydrates below 50 grams per day, and following my 2-2-2-2 rule for healing fat intake.

- Choose **two** days this week to fast—either a complete fast, a partial (500-800 calories and protein under 15-20 grams) or consume one regular low-carb meal and eat to full. If you feel you are not yet ready for a full twenty-four hour fast, you can consume coconut oil or MCT oil during the day or with your morning coffee, but test as described in Chapter 3, to help increase your fast adaptation and prepare you to fast next week fully. The choice of the partial fast of 500–800 calories and keeping protein under 15–20 grams a day is amazing for gaining more autophagy during your fast days. These fasting days should not be back-to-back but separated.

- One day of the week is a fun "carb-load" or "protein-load" day. The carb-load day serves to refill your glycogen stores and reminds your body that it is not starving. The protein-load day seems to work better for some of my clients, especially those with certain gut issues. We can also alter load days every other week (one week carb-load, the following week protein-load, and so forth), depending on what works best for your body, health goals, and conditions.

4-2-1 Weekly Example

FOUR days of regular intermittent fasting/ keto. Eat a ketogenic diet and check your blood ketones to make sure you're in ketosis. During these 4 days, follow the 2-2-2-2 rule:

- Add 2 Tbs. MCT or coconut oil

- Add 2 Tbs. high quality salt

- Add 2 Tbs. grass fed organic butter

- Add 2 Tbs. Olive Oil

- Intermittent fast 15-18 hours

TWO days of complete or partial fasting (the famine day). Choose:

- Water fast all day

- One meal a day (eat to satiety). 22-24 hour dinner-to-dinner or breakfast-to-breakfast fasts.

- Partial fasting: 500-800 calories and under 20 grams of protein. Eat in small window, around 6 hours.

ONE day of increased carbohydrate OR increased protein (the feast day). Eat up to 100-200 grams of healthy carbs OR protein). The carb (or protein) load day serves to refill your glycogen stores, and reminds your body that it is not starving.

- Pick one day where you (with intention) eat more. Focus on increasing your carbohydrate (OR protein) intake particularly.

- Choose carbohydrates from nutrient-dense sources like sweet potatoes, yams, fruit, or ancient grains. Carbs (or protein) up to around 100-200 grams to remind the body that it isn't starving.

SAMPLE 4-2-1 FEAST/FAMINE CYCLING MEAL PLAN

You have worked hard to this point, so take some time to acknowledge where you are in the process. Maybe you are still not fat adapted, but well on your way, or feeling amazing and adapted quickly. Regardless of where you are in your journey, take time to reflect upon your successes, however big or small. Making big dietary changes is difficult, and we hope step-by- step we have taken things at a good pace for you, preparing you for next week, the five-day fast, whichever fast you choose.

NOTE: Italicized items can be found in the *Meal Plans and Recipes* section.

Monday: Famine Day

Meal 1 (3 pm): *Omelet* with spinach, parsley, leeks, arugula, and avocado; Optional: Bacon or shredded chicken

Tuesday

Meal 1 (2 pm): *Coconut Wraps* with sardines, avocado, cucumber, and parsley

Meal 2 (6 pm): Big green salad, with beef, tomatoes avocado, olive oil, and lemon juice

Wednesday

Meal 1 (2 pm): *Green Soup* topped with bacon bits and avocado

Meal 2 (6 pm): Oven-baked salmon with roasted fennel and carrots

Thursday: Famine Day

Meal 1 (Noon): *Creamy Chocolate Avocado Smoothie*

Friday

Meal 1 (2 pm): *Oven-Baked Crispy, Spicy Chicken Wings* with raw carrots, celery, and a blue cheese dip

Meal 2 (6 pm): Big green salad, with beef, tomatoes, avocado, olive oil, and lemon juice

Saturday: Feast Day

Meal 1 (2 pm): *Banana Pancakes with Coconut Yogurt and Cinnamon*

Meal 2 (6 pm): *Sweet Potato "Toast"* with avocado, smoked salmon

Sunday

Meal 1 (2 pm): Roasted asparagus soup with olive oil and crumbled feta

Meal 2 (6 pm): Curry chicken on a bed of greens

THE FIVE-DAY WATER FAST

*I*MPORTANT NOTE: If you have health challenges or a known health condition, you should work with one of our Platinum Health Centers of the Future Doctors trained in this entire program. Always check with your doctor before starting any new health program or fast.

You have already gone beyond fasting and learned the lifestyle my wife and I live, not just to maximize the results of a fast, but to maximize our lives. With the three to four five-day fasts a year and all you have put into action; you have added healthy years to your life. We both have measured this with telomere testing, which measures the length of your telomeres (the best indicator of your biological age). Accurate testing can help determine your cellular biological age versus your actual age.

My first cellular age test reflected at 11 years older than my actual age, and now I am 10 years younger than my actual age. My wife is far younger, fortunately, and unfortunately for me. She is 30 years of age at the cellular level. The test doesn't accurately go below age 30. Therefore, I could be married to a 20-year-old at this point. Not sure if that is good or bad! Ha! You have trained for this fast as you would train for a race. Your results will be amazing regardless of which fast you choose.

If water fasting scares you too much, fear not. There are two other choices explained here as well; a partial fast and what is known as the *Fasting Mimicking Diet™*.

I have been teaching fasting for a long time, to both clients and doctors. Many of these doctors give me feedback from the different fasts, and we noticed that something magical happened around Day 4, where the body transitions into this amazing fat-burning machine. We also see this increase in stem cells,[1] and then on Day 5, even more so.[2]

Clinically, we recommend a four-day minimum. The first three days, you are just breaking through the loss of hunger and using fat and ketones for energy. The body is revving up the autophagy. The hormones are adjusting, and growth hormone is starting to rise.[3] On Day 4, people tend to stop feeling hungry and get a sudden burst of energy. We want people to ride that for one more day, and science backs up the big rise in growth hormone and stem cells on Day 5. In Week 7, you will learn why the refeed on Day 6 for feeding these new stem cells is so important. So, hang in there—you will get to eat!

Fasting is one of my ancient healing strategies in the multi-therapeutic approach I teach, and I honestly believe it works miracles for people. Fasting has changed the lives of many of my clients and has improved my health and that of my family. However, it is not something you want to take on without having a strategic plan in place, especially water fasting, which requires experienced hands and minds to guide you through safely to get the best results. Therefore, we have doctors and practitioners trained to assist for a safe and more effective fast. If you have challenges, perhaps a partial fast or a Fasting Mimicking Diet described later in this chapter would be suitable places to start.

THE SEVEN ACCOMPLISHMENTS OF FASTING

1. Autophagy

Autophagy, or self-eating, is the process by which the body naturally removes cellular debris, meaning the body will always eat the bad cells and tissues for energy before using the good ones. Bad cells cannot adapt to using fat for energy, so they die off and become food for the body.[4]

This process is important because it's these bad cells that could lead to a variety of health ailments in the body, including:

- Increased inflammation which is a causative factor in most degenerative diseases and why most people don't feel well.

- Food allergies and intolerances

- Autoimmune diseases—rheumatoid arthritis, lupus, celiac disease, cancer.

- Diabetes and thyroid conditions

- Weight loss resistance

- Autism, Alzheimer's, and other neurodegenerative diseases

- Many studies show fasting can turn down an overactive immune system responsible for these conditions,[5] and has also been shown to regenerate pancreatic cells, and in animal models can even reverse diabetes. It does this by "recycling" the bad cells (autophagy) to fuel new stem cell production for cellular "renewal."

2. Stem Cells

Stem cells are unspecialized cells that give rise to differentiated cells. They are often called "master cells" because they can grow into any of the body's 200 types of cells.[7] What many people don't realize is there is a rise in stem cells during and after a fast, so this explains many of the miraculous healings that occur with fasting.[8]

According to a recent study by Italian researcher Valter Longo, prolonged fasting breaks down a significant amount of white blood cells. During each cycle of fasting, this depletion of white blood cells induces changes that trigger stem cell-based regeneration of new immune system cells.[9]

Most times, older cells the body used were the over-reactive cells that would lead to autoimmunity (hyperimmunity) and other health issues as described in the earlier section. Thanks to the regeneration of newer, younger cells in the body, a better functioning immune system is possible. Clinically we see this amazing result that truly transforms lives.

One of the amazing experiences during a fast is the random pains in areas of past injuries or areas that need healing. The pain or discomfort felt is most often because of the autophagy stem cell reaction going on in that area of the body. Some would call this re-tracing, where the body goes back to old symptoms or injuries as part of the healing process. Science could never explain the phenomenon so many described during fasting or detox, but I believe the new science and studies will soon give us the answer.

People pay much money for stem cell injections today for incredible regeneration of joints and to anti-age, and many times they need it. Fortunately, the best news of all is the body will make them for free during a fast.

3. **Ketones**

Burning fat cells for energy produces ketones, which help to down- regulate cellular inflammation, heal the gut, and heal the brain. Ketones can also turn off bad genes and turn on good ones that help us live longer, healthier lives.[10]

When you do an extended fast, your body will use the ketones because it must live. After approximately three days of fasting, the body adapts to using these ketones, and the levels are far higher than when in ketosis alone without a fasting state. As a result, the health benefits from ketones are much greater.[11]

During ketosis diets, the ketones do not get as high as needed for the amazing healing that we see in studies. During fasting, we see ketones four times as high on average than with a ketosis diet alone. Another benefit of the fasting ketones is that they are in the presence of low glucose. Thomas Seyfried, the famous cancer researcher and author of, *Cancer as a Metabolic Disease*, states you do not get the benefits of ketones without a drop in glucose.

4. **Energy Diversion**

One of the most important (and overlooked) aspects of fasting is energy diversion. Energy diversion is the description of what happens during our fast to cause healing of old injuries or damaged organs.

Many of us do not understand how much energy it takes to metabolize food. You may think, "Okay, I'm just eating, and obviously, there's some energy output here." That's true, but then the body must digest it, which takes massive energy. Then it must assimilate it, which requires the greatest amount of energy. Next, we have what happens at the cell level. The body takes that energy and drives all these processes from glycolysis to the Krebs cycle - massive ATP use, massive energy output. The more energy you burn or use, the more pollution you create (endogenous toxins), which is another energy output to clean up the pollution and down-regulate that inflammation and oxidative stress. We're demanding the body's massive energy output digest and assimilate food rather than go towards healing. Here's the point: When we stop eating, the body goes, "Wait a minute: what am I going to do with all this energy?"

It's like when you have time off work, you have nothing specific planned and may wonder what you will do with all that extra time and energy. Guess what the body does? It doesn't sit back on the couch and watch TV. Instead, it says, "I will put that energy to healing." It's energy diversion, so it shifts the energy used when eating to healing the body.

You have heard me say I tell my clients: "Don't eat less; eat less often." When we looked at the studies, we thought, "Oh, eating less is the key to living longer." Technically, it is, but the key is to eat less by eating less often. By not eating throughout the day, your body uses that energy for better processes of healing. It's merely diverting that energy to repair the body. During five-day fasts, much of the pain we get in those old injured areas is the body using its newfound energy to go back and heal. The body knew this organ or tissue needed healing, but it was simply prioritizing the energy for daily survival and not for healing.

5. Hormone Optimization

Even during a short fast, there's a rapid increase in growth hormone and especially Day 5 of a five-day fast. However, perfecting hormones is not just about gaining more hormones, but about becoming more hormone sensitive. Hormones like testosterone and growth hormone, or any that affect healing, dramatically amp up during a fast to hold on to your muscle for survival, but the cells become extremely sensitive to the hormones.[12] If your cells hear the hormones better, this means you feel better.

Over time with more fasting, our cells become increasingly sensitive to our hormones, even insulin. For example, during a fast, hormone sensitivity increases for insulin and thyroid hormone to burn your fat and to spare its muscle. Again, it's all about survival[13] and using the hormone optimization for the adaptation. If the body doesn't adapt, it dies; it's that simple.

With each fast, the body becomes more hormonally optimized, and the more metabolically flexible you become (better at burning fat) and the healthier you become.

6. Reset Microbiome: Gut Bacteria

Fasting will repair the gut barrier. Environmental changes and stressors have been shown to change the microbiome, which can have a dramatic effect on gut healing.[14] Fasting is especially restorative for a leaky gut, described as when the intestine wall shows excessive permeability and linked to autoimmune and other unexplainable illnesses. Fasting provides a break from digesting food, allowing the body time to "heal and seal" the gut lining. I've seen fasts heal serious gut conditions repeatedly, which is critical because over 80% of your immunity lies in the gut, and the microbiome influences our genetic expression. Fasting starves out bad bacteria, and refeeding with fermented foods helps to repopulate the gut with beneficial bacteria. The doctors I coach, and I, all agree that you don't fix a bad gut with probiotics, but you can with the fasting strategies in this book. Part of the gut healing also comes from certain autoimmune genes being turned off during the fast leading to #7.[16]

7. Resets DNA Gene Code

The last benefit of fasting pertains to our DNA.[17] Recently, several studies have come out saying something I have instinctively known for years: People didn't get sick from their bad genes, but from bad lifestyles and living in a toxic world.

One thing I learned from this research is that you can have the best protocol, diet, and intentions, but if a bad gene of susceptibility turns on and expresses an unhealthy condition, it must be turned off for true healing and a lasting change.[18] Today, when we hear the term "it runs in my family," that normally means genetics, where genes pass from the parents to their children, generation to generation. This comment leads people to believe that most sickness transfers down through the generations and there is not much they can do about it.[19]

Thankfully, this is not true in most cases. Thanks to the new science of epigenetics, we have discovered we can now free ourselves from the diseases that may have plagued our families for generations. For example, a doctor may say to you that you have high blood pressure because your mom has it.[20] They told me this when I was in the ninth grade. Today, I have normal blood pressure. Through my cellular detox and fasting, I have turned off this gene. Your DNA is not your destiny, especially when you incorporate fasting into your life.

Genetics do not affect our thoughts and feelings either, our environment, and how we react to it does. When the mind experiences feelings like stress and fear, it protects itself by releasing chemicals that get us ready for fight or flight. Fight or flight means I will use my arms and legs. I've got to run away, or I've got to fight. What do the hormones and chemicals of fear do? They shut down all the mechanisms of the body that have nothing to do with protection, to distribute all the energy of the body for protection.[21] Then we become genetically stuck in a stress response mode. It's called sympathetic dominance. This state can cause disease.

Even though the body is in a constant state of stress and energy is being diverted to the perceived danger, it still must replace billions of cells every day. These billions of new cells are invariably weaker than the cells they are replacing, thus lowering the body's immune system, and increasing the susceptibility to illness and disease.[22] We can change this stress state by downregulating the triggered genes that keep this reaction going. Fasting has been shown to turn off these genes and is like stress reset.[24]

Fasting goes beyond these seven accomplishments. There are so many more benefits that science has yet to discover. We are only now able to explain scientifically some of the miracles we see during a fast. However, I can tell you from years of observation that there is so much more that takes place when you allow the innate intelligence of the body to find homeostasis, healing balance.

LESSONS FROM OLYMPIC GOLD MEDALIST, TORAH BRIGHT

One of my clients, Torah Bright, is an Australian professional snowboarder and Australia's most successful Winter Olympian and a former Olympic gold and silver medalist, who took her healing to the next level through a five-day water fast. She had a history of brain trauma, which can create an environment for more toxins to enter the brain. Torah fasted for five days. She shared her fasting story with me, admitting that she had been a bit nervous about taking it on. However, she went into her fast already in a state of ketosis, using intermittent daily fasting and the diet variation principles described in this program.

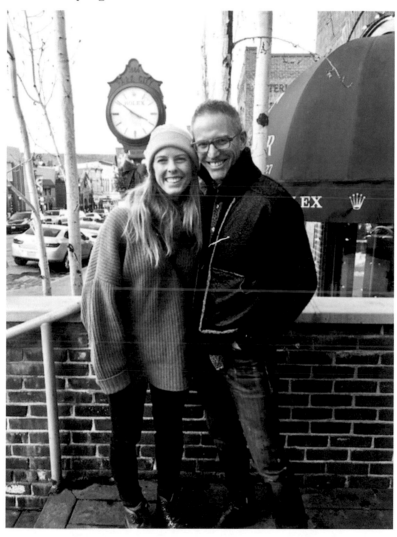

The first two days were rough for Torah mentally, and the third day was the most challenging. On the third day, she felt the most tired and sore, as old injuries were healing. On Day 4 Torah said that she woke up and felt amazing. Overall, fasting was key to bringing Torah's healing to the next level in her brain, and she loved the experience. She could go back into the competition but afterward realized there was so much more she wanted to do besides compete. At least she had the chance and choice to do so. It's important to point out she had tried everything and saw the best doctors, but in this case, like so many, the best doctor was to be found within.

Torah said, "When I broke the fast and got into food again, it was a spiritual experience for me. It was a calming, healing, spiritual experience. I loved it, and I can't wait to do another one." Torah has done many fasts now and has become proficient at all techniques in this book, including cellular detox.

LESSONS FROM DR. POMPA'S DAUGHTER, OLIVIA MAKE SURE YOUR TEENAGERS READ THIS

"Fasting has been part of my daily lifestyle for the past six to seven years. I began experimenting on myself during high school, with guidance from my father, Dr. Daniel Pompa, a fasting and ketogenic guru. I committed to a lifestyle of "eating less often" by choice to improve my health early in my adult life and to have a personal testimony about such a controversial topic.

I experienced my first car accident around the age of 18. At some point, I lost control, and I flew off the road, tumbled a few times and landed upside down in panic mode. I quickly unbuckled my seat belt to crawl out of the passenger side window, smacking my head on the roof of the car. I am thankful to have walked away from this accident with only a minor concussion. However, what is most important is that complications arising after the accident led to the diagnosis of inner-lying health issues.

From that day forward, I experienced an odd, unexplainable pressure in my head, and in my best description, it was almost like a constant drunk feeling, but now I know it was "brain fog." I was struggling to focus in school, and the inability to feel present day-to-day was making me angry. I went through concussion treatment at a renowned university neurology center in Atlanta, GA, to help fix what I thought was post-concussion syndrome. This process did not help in the slightest, not because the treatment was insufficient, but because I was suffering from underlying toxicity, and the symptoms I was experiencing were unexplainable from a diagnosing doctor's standpoint.

I began undergraduate work at Florida State University, and studied in Spain my first year, where I had the freedom to make those famous bad decisions, ending up with another concussion one evening after smacking my head on a dance floor. I went to the hospital for treatment, and the doctors urged me to take the medications for headaches, nausea, and dizziness. This time, I would not accept that the symptoms would "heal over time" because I knew that the brain fog would only get worse.

So, this is where my fasting journey truly begins. My father, being a fasting guru, urged fasting for five days, convincing me it would speed up the healing process in my brain. When I woke up on the sixth day and had my first small "meal," within a few hours, my head was clearer than it had been in months. It felt like a miracle. My energy improved, my brain fog was gone, and during that month, I rarely experienced any headaches. It became clear to me that fasting was something special, and more individuals my age needed to try it.

Okay, so who is fasting these days, and why?

Fasting is an ancient healing practice, so it has been around for a long time and is still used among many religious groups. Today, aside from the spiritual intent, eating in time windows has become popular among bodybuilders, those with diabetes, autoimmune disorders, obesity, and those on a search for best mind and body wellness. I'll catch your attention with this one: Many are using fasting even to prevent or reverse cancer. It's interesting to me that without food, your body can heal itself as was intended, without the use of human-made drugs. Sounds possible, right?

During the long-term fasted state, the body produces ketones from metabolizing fat as a source of fuel, a crucial adaptation as the brain's major source of fuel is glucose (or carbohydrates). However, in times of starvation or famine when carbohydrates are unavailable, the brain can metabolically switch from using glucose to using ketones for energy. I'd say that's neat.

Ketones burn cleaner than glucose, so, using ketones produces less inflammation and oxidative stress; preventing damage to other cells. Research shows ketone use increases growth hormone, reduces inflammation and its markers, repairs mitochondria, regulates hormones, increases good cholesterol, and decreases bad, regulates blood sugar, improves cognitive function, and the list continues. These benefits are why many are using fasting to reverse a condition or to perfect wellness. I believe fasting is the only "medicine" America needs.

As a young adult in college, I believe we should educate other young adults about preventative health, and this goes beyond eating healthy and exercising. Today's young adults are far from healthy. It's common to assume that young bodies can recover from years of heavy drinking, drugs, and constant stress. As we examine the health of my generation, it is scary to see how health issues we commonly see in adults are already creeping up on and progressing in my friends. Brain fog is popular among my generation, and most are quickly prescribed study drugs to keep up with the other stimulated students in their schools. However, it's okay because they are prescribed and "needed," right?

Wrong.

Their inability to focus in school is a cognitive dysfunction; it's not normal. My brother has ADHD, has never been medicated and uses fasting to improve his cognitive function, as do I. In fact, the more I fast, the better are my ability and focus in school. My mind has become clear, and with an unclouded mind, I feel limitless. My generation has the power and the resources to educate themselves and those around them on preventative medicine, including the extensive benefits of natural healing such as fasting.

I want to spread the excitement about ketosis and fasting to my generation, and this inspiration has, of course, come from my testimony and improvement in mental and physical wellness, but also from the testimonies of my friends whose lives are progressively improving. Preventative health is exciting, and it is crucial if we want to see our young adults and college students thrive in this world more than we have ever seen before."

IMPORTANT: Everyone can benefit from undertaking a fast. Keep in mind, if it is a water fast only you are choosing, it is water only. What does this mean for you? Only drink water. No tea. No coffee. No supplements (there may be exceptions to this as you will see). Nothing but water, and a little sea salt - GOOD sea salt like pink Himalayan.

MY SPIRITUAL PERSPECTIVE ABOUT FASTING

Every major religious group on the planet promotes fasting for a purpose. Fasting is the only thing about which every religious group agrees even if they do not agree on prayer practices. We fast to become more connected and aware spiritually, emotionally, and even physically to "something" outside of ourselves. We hear stories and testimonies of breakthroughs through fasting. Even ideas and creative thoughts that have been swirling in the brain without direction have come together through fasting. We have personally experienced all these things and more. We have noted that emotional clarity can stabilize our feelings and perspectives, which holds tremendous value if emotionally connected to a situation.

From the spiritual perspective, I can share a personal story of our son, who was being led astray and causing us great distress. We are not willing to share all the details, as many of them would seem unbelievable without in-depth conversation and without having been there to see it. However, what I will share is that God woke my wife during the night with a simple word: "FAST," and she at once did. Five days later, a layer of that oppression fled. With each fast since, and there have been two, and soon a third, the enemy is fleeing.

We are relentless in our prayer for the continuation of God's hand upon the situation and the culmination of His purposes within it, but we are doing our part, and we know He will do His. While we may not always understand why we can have certain experiences, we do understand that as our faith grows, we can look back and know we would not be who we are without these experiences. I have experienced many breakthroughs each time I have fasted. Some things have had more meaning than others, but all things have proven requests we have made to God.

My wife added this accompanying scripture to her fast and continues to this day to remind not just herself but many others: "But this kind does not go out except by prayer and fasting." Matthew 17:21. Since this time, we now understand firsthand how much value there is to prayer and fasting for our children.

I never expect everyone to believe as I believe, but I think this will still encourage all of us. My favorite Bible chapter about the power of fasting is, 2 Chronicles 20, especially if you are going through a very challenging time. When we are facing something much bigger than we can manage this will empower you and give you hope.

In this chapter of the Bible, there was a vast army made up of three different nations who were coming against Israel. In great fear, King Jehoshaphat inquired of the Lord and "proclaimed a fast for all Judah."

This is what the Lord says to you: Do not be afraid or discouraged because of this vast army. For the battle is not yours, but God's.16 Tomorrow march down against them. They will be climbing up by the Pass of Ziz, and you will find them at the end of the gorge in the Desert of Jeruel.17 You will not have to fight this battle. Take up your positions; stand firm and see the deliverance the Lord will give you, Judah, and Jerusalem. Do not be afraid; do not be discouraged. Go out to face them tomorrow, and the Lord will be with you.

What this chapter of scripture anchors me to is that regardless of my "battles" whether physical or emotional, God has won the battle for me, just as He has for you, and fasting is the surrender to demonstrating to Him with an act of my will that I trust Him with it. After all, He desires children that respond to Him in love, just as we do as earthly parents with our children.

After the battle, Israel gathered the plunder, and the Bible says there was "...so much plunder that it took three days to collect." 2 Chronicles 20:25.

In our case, the plunder was our son. What will yours be?

WEIGHT LOSS: ANOTHER SIDE BENEFIT

Another consideration when fasting is rapid weight loss. When carefully executed, water fasting can help tremendously with fat loss [25] and uprooting deep toxins stored in the tissue.[26] However, weight loss is not the primary goal for everyone who partakes in a fast. As stated already, weight gain is another benefit. The innate intelligence knows this and seeks balance (homeostasis). The body knows how to eat damaged tissue and bad DNA (autophagy) while routinely avoiding muscle.[27] This situation is marvelous for tumors—the body will eat those too.

It is a myth that fasting lowers your metabolism. It's the opposite, it raises your metabolism to survive on its fat, and it optimizes its hormones to keeps its muscle to survive, which also stimulates the metabolism. Caloric restriction long term, as mentioned earlier, lowers metabolism for the same reason—to survive. It will stop burning fat because it thinks it's starving and wants to hang on to its only fuel, happening only after a prolonged time of caloric restriction. Therefore, partial fasting with five days of caloric restriction, and water fasting for five days work because those fasts are not long enough to kick in the starvation mode. That mode takes many days and months for most people. Caloric restriction long term also fails because the hunger hormone ghrelin keeps rising, causing hunger never to stop, unlike a fast, where ghrelin drops and stabilizes typically causing the hunger to go away by Day 3.

You will lose on average one half to one pound a day during a water fast and slightly less with a partial or Fasting Mimicking Diet. However, fasting will kick in the hormone optimization needed for continued weight loss even after the fast is over. Recall that the cells become more insulin sensitive with each fast and studies show this continues beyond the fast if continuing with the dietary changes. The principles of *Beyond Fasting*, when done throughout the year, are the real keys to continue weight loss and hormone optimization.

LOW IMMUNITY, HYPERIMMUNITY (FOOD ALLERGIES AND SENSITIVITIES) AND AUTOIMMUNITY

We used to think fasting lowered the immune system because of lower amounts of white blood cells during a fast. With new research, we have learned that the opposite is true. The body has an innate intelligence and knows to eat the bad or overactive immune cells first. It's these bad cells that drive inflammation and hyperimmunity seen in allergies, food sensitivities,[17] and autoimmune disorders.[18] The older cells that have been around too long become hypersensitive, driving the inflammation that's responsible for most of the conditions affecting millions of people.[19]

When people say, "I just don't feel well," and have had many tests done that turn out negative, this can be part of the reason. It can take up to thirty years of this hyperimmune state before getting a diagnosis of an autoimmune condition. Testing for autoimmune conditions is still very much in the early phases, so this possibility could be why you don't feel well.

Valter Longo is an Italian American biogerontologist and cell biologist known for his studies on the role of fasting and nutrient response genes on cellular protection, aging, and diseases, and for proposing that similar genes and mechanisms in many cells regulate longevity. His research shows that the immune system repairs and gets stronger during a fast. Yes, white blood cells drop, but this is because of autophagy, and the rise in stem cells makes new, more naïve immune cells that do not overreact creating inflammation.

Fasting Healed My Hashimoto Diagnosis

Five years ago, at age 36, I was diagnosed with Hashimoto's - an autoimmune disease that targets the thyroid. As a result, my thyroid was underactive, and my antibodies commonly ranged from 900-1200 iu/mL across several lab tests. To remedy this, I tried taking thyroid supplements, and then Armour® Thyroid and ended up resorting to prescription T3 (liothyronine). During this time, I was losing hair, gaining weight, and suffering from fatigue and chronic constipation. I was already eating a clean diet, exercising, and working on my health pre-diagnosis, but it seemed that no matter what I did, my health was refusing to budge.

Then I found *Cellular Healing TV*. Dr. Pompa spoke about detox, fasting, and even had an episode on Hashimoto's - I was blown away. I will never forget the first time I watched him draw the cell and explain why everything I was trying was not working. I immediately started intermittent fasting multiple times a week and slowly worked my way up to 24-48 hour fasts. I noticed a major difference in my digestive health with just this small change to my lifestyle. For the last three years, I have adhered to what Dr. Pompa teaches; I started True Cellular Detox, got my amalgams removed, finished TCD, and completed multiple Brain Phases. I also do 3 to 4 five-day water fasts a year along with partial fasts, intermittent fasts, regular 24-hour fasts. The last step I took to combat my Hashimoto's was to have my cavitations removed in August of 2018. I re-tested my labs 6 months after cavitation removal and my thyroid numbers were normal for the first time in years. Wow!

This was accomplished by following Dr. Pompa's Multi Therapeutic Approach without even targeting my thyroid; instead, I went upstream, and I targeted the things that made my thyroid off balance.

WHAT IF I AM UNDERWEIGHT AND
DON'T WANT TO LOSE MUSCLE?

Alongside the weight loss, there may also be some who need weight gain or who fear losing muscle. With the rapid healing of the gut, hormone optimization, and the rise in stem cells, the fast can be a strategic tool for gaining muscle.[28] Growth hormone and testosterone increase during both short fasts and extended fasts.[29,30]

The YouTube sensation, the Hodge twins, undertake on an average sixteen to nineteen-hour fasts most days, powered by an eight to five-hour feeding period. They do take in lots of calories and protein in this window to help in muscle growth; however, they credited this fast as a critical part of their process for bodybuilding.

Even extended fasting is an amazing strategy for gaining muscle. I hear people say, "I can't fast because I am so underweight." However, after a month or two post fast, the body will gain muscle weight because of autophagy/stem cell activity. During the fast, the body loses some muscle (protein) via autophagy, but it is only the bad protein or muscle that is not healthy and is not recovering from exercise. The stem cells rise after the fast brings new muscle cells that are healthy and adapt to the exercise and become stronger and fuller.

Recall that I challenged my middle son Izik to this because he was afraid to fast thinking he would lose muscle. He lost about twelve pounds during his fast and ended up a month later gaining that back plus eight more pounds of muscle. I see this in clients all the time. Even better digestion and assimilation of food post fast play a critical role in quality weight gain for those who are sick and challenged.

My wife Merily credits her multiple water-only fasts to her muscle gain and the leanest she has ever been in her life, and she is in her 50s. I show pictures of her in the gym in my lecture to prove that the muscle loss during a fast is a myth and in fact, it's the opposite.

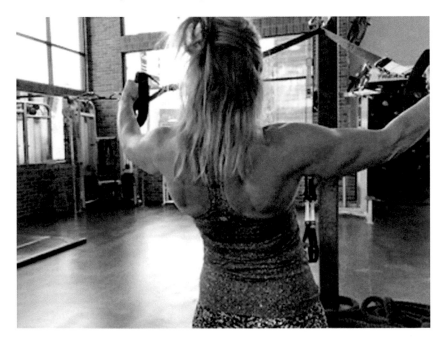

IMPORTANT NOTE: If you are on medications, continue your medications. If you wish to change a dose or stop a certain medication, it's important that you consult with your doctor on this.

HOW DO I WATER FAST?

If you choose a water fast, the protocol is quite simple. Drink when you're thirsty. There is no need to drink water all day if you are not thirsty or consume a certain predetermined amount of water each day. Drinking too much water can overstress the kidneys. You can add a little pink Himalayan salt for minerals, and to help keep hunger at bay. It's unnecessary, but some people find it helpful to do so, especially if you are new to fasting.

WHAT IF I MESS UP MY FAST BY EATING SOMETHING?

If you break from the fast, or "mess up" when you are not through the five days yet, it's okay. Just breath, get back on track, and continue pushing forward. Don't let that be a reason to quit.

Three reasons you might not feel well, and some solutions:

1. **Low electrolytes:** Add sea salt to your water to help support electrolytes. Taking magnesium may help some (I recommend magnesium malate or magnesium glycinate), or you may need to take a stronger, more balanced electrolyte-just find one without sugar.

2. **Not be fully fat adapted:** You may need to spend more time in the earlier steps or more variation in the diet weekly or monthly (see Weeks 4 and 5).

3. **Still not fat adapted even following this protocol?** You may struggle with some neurotoxicity. I recommend our "fasting trio," CytoDetox®, BIND, and Fastonic. However, some may have deep toxic issues and need one of our Platinum doctors trained in Cellular Detox.

   - **Fastonic** down-regulates hydroxy free radicals—free radicals cause inflammation and unwanted symptoms, especially during fasting.

- **BIND** prevents the toxins from the gut to recirculate back into the body (auto-intoxication), leading to many unwanted symptoms.

- **CytoDetox®** helps support the body in the toxin elimination from the cells.

THE PARTIAL FAST: ANOTHER OPTION

The best choice for a fast is the one you don't fear, and with which you will stick. I will say from my clinical experience; we see the greatest breakthroughs from water fasting, where you can receive the maximum benefits of autophagy and stem cell production. However, I will give some of you a little bailout here that will still yield amazing results and sometimes better results. There is a fast I have used for years known as "the partial fast."

The partial fast, like the Fasting Mimicking Diet that I will discuss next, involves cutting caloric and protein intake during the day for the period of the fast (not long-term). I prefer five days. We can also do these fasts five days every month with ease. We should not mix up this type of fasting with juice fasting, of which I am not a fan. There are many clinical situations where I favor partial fasting over water only, and the results for these people and conditions are better. If you are not breaking through in fat adaptation (ketosis) or struggling with intermittent fasting, then I would say that is a clue that this is a better place to start.

NOTE: If you have health challenges and no supervision, then this or the Fasting Mimicking Diet (ProLon Fast) would be a safer place to start, but always check with your doctor before starting any new health program or fast as the medication will need to be adjusted.

For a partial fast, cut calories to 500–1000 per day, 500–700 for smaller individuals (100–150 lbs.). Larger people (150–200 lbs.) would consume 700–900 calories. Anyone above 200 pounds should consume 900–1100 calories per day. It's a low protein (under 15–20 grams a day), high fat and low-carbohydrate, and no meat diet. With partial fasting, stick with simple foods. The focus is on eating vegetables and fats. During a partial fast, my 2-2-2-2 rule is the main caloric sources you are taking in. We can hit 500 calories very quickly. For example, one tablespoon of oil has 120 calories. Bone broth is another reliable source of calories, and it feels nice to have something warm to sip.

Decreased calories and decreased protein are proven to stimulate autophagy. With the partial fast, you get many of the same benefits you would from a water fast. For some people, it's difficult to do a water fast. Partial fasting gives these individuals another choice. That you get to eat a little bit in the day may be helpful for some people. You can consume the calories in either one or two meals within that eating window. For some people who are fearful of a water fast, this is a good option.

What are some health benefits associated with partial fasting?

- Lowered calorie and protein intake mimics fasting and reboots the body.[31]

- Promotes autophagy (removal of cellular debris) for healthy mitochondria and longevity.[32]

- Helps to decrease inflammation and rest digestion.[33]

- It kick-starts weight loss.[34]

- Easier for some to follow than traditional fasting.

- Helpful for those with low nutritional stores who seek fasting benefits.

When are the best times to partake in partial fasting?

- Five days a month for several months to build on the autophagy and stem cell activation.

- After a water or broth fast to continue benefits and transition to solid foods.

- For diet variation: Do one to three random days weekly (rotate days for variation, for example, Tuesday and Thursday).

- For deeper cellular repair: Do longer (five to ten days) partial fast monthly or seasonally.

Basics and Rules of Engagement:

- Use with an intermittent fasting style of eating approximately one to two meals within a compressed time window.

- Consume 500–1100 calories daily for health benefits.

- Base daily calorie goals on body weight for best results. (See below)

- Foods should fall into categories of fat, fiber, fruits, and vegetables to cover nutritional needs.

- Partial fast can include only liquid, in the form of smoothies and shakes, to rest the digestive system.

- Protein shouldn't exceed 15–20 grams a day to avoid shutting down autophagy.

- Consume adequate good fat to maintain satiety and blood sugar.

- Consume most calories during the early afternoon to early evening (1– 6 pm), but meal timing can vary.

- Use online food calculators to check calories and macros.

- Gentle exercise (walking, yoga) is acceptable during partial fasting; we do not recommend intense exercise, especially for those with health changes.

- Supplements can be continued, unlike water fasting.

NOTE: *Medications should be continued but check with your doctor for possible adjustment throughout the fast.*

CALORIES BASED ON BODY WEIGHT

Approximate Weight	Approximate Daily Calorie Intake
100–150 lbs.	500–700
150–200 lbs.	700–900
200 lbs. or more	900–1100

FOUR BASIC CATEGORIES AND WHOLE FOOD EXAMPLES FOR PARTIAL FASTING

- Choose two to four servings from each food category daily (depending on the caloric goal).

- Consume one half to one whole avocado daily.

- Consume one half to one cup of berries daily.

- Choose organic when possible.

The chart offers basic ranges; calculate calories for accuracy. 500–700 calories: Approximately two servings from each group. 700–900 calories: Approximately three servings from each group. 900–1100 calories: Approximately four servings from each group.

FAT (Oils) Choose 2-4 (1 Tbs. each)	FIBER (Nuts and seeds) Choose 2-4 (2 Tbs. each)	FRUIT Choose 2-4 (½-1 cup)	VEGETABLES Choose 2-4 (1-3 cups)
• Coconut oil, butter, or flakes • Olive oil • Grass-fed butter or butter oil • Macadamia nut oil • MCT oil • Avocado oil • Hemp oil • Flax oil	• Chia seed • Flaxseed • Tiger nuts, flour, flakes • Hemp seeds • Raw nuts and seeds • Macadamia nuts, pumpkin seeds, if no allergy	• Blueberries • Raspberries • Strawberries • Blackberries • Avocado	• Leafy greens • Broccoli • Cauliflower • Brussels Sprouts • Artichokes • Carrots • Sweet Potato • Squash

If you do not feel ready to start with a full-out fast, partial fasting makes for a great transitional choice. With that said, I recommend working your way up to a full five days or longer fast. In doing so, you will experience the maximum benefits fasting has to offer.

FASTING MIMICKING DIET™ THIS FAST MAKES IT EASY WITH PROVEN RESULTS.

Valter Longo is doing new research and is the developer of the *Fasting Mimicking Diet™* and a fasting product called ProLon. Like a partial fast, the calories are cut to 500-1000 calories and protein to under 20 grams per day for five days. However, he has scientifically dialed in the amounts of protein, carbs, and fats for maximizing the results. He holds the patent on this formula, and because he is the brains behind so many new studies coming out and has recently received over forty million dollars from the NIH in grants for new studies, he may have a superior product and formula for what he would say is the perfect fast.

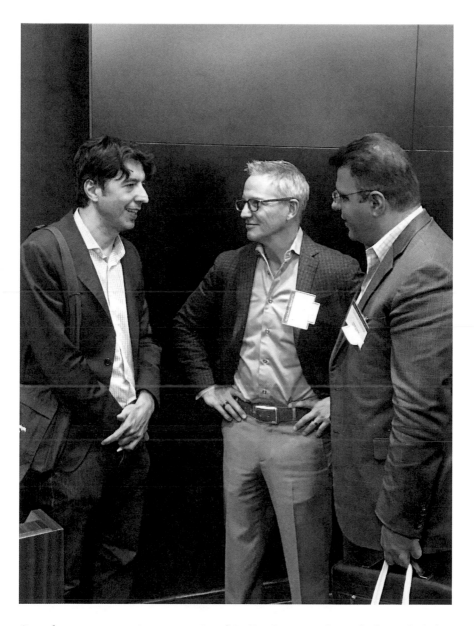

Our doctor group is now using his ProLon product (a boxed 5-day fast) in some of our fasts replacing the use of the partial fast we have used for years. The ProLon is a scientifically developed box of food for each day of the five-day fast. Each box has Longo's patented ratios. He says there are volumes of research that have gone into why these specific foods maximize the results and safety. I can say this: The boxed food makes it easy to be compliant, "Here is what I have to eat today." It worked for Nutrisystem and Jenny Craig, so there is something to the compliance aspect.

I think it is a safe and great fast to start with, especially for those with metabolic challenges or don't have a doctor to check your fast. ProLon has people to help in this area and even get questions answered. We have found this fast, successful, and simple for people to do.

A recent animal study from Valter Longo and his group showed five days of a fast emulating the ProLon Fasting Mimicking Diet for five consecutive months regenerated beta cells in the pancreas of mice. This study is groundbreaking because it shows the power of autophagy and stem cell activation via fasting. It also illustrates the power of this type of fasting. With the money granted from the NIH, there are over twenty studies in progress, with some repetition using human subjects and with the potential to change health care and the state of degenerative disease in this country. The studies are critical to legitimize fasting and what we have seen for years with the power of fasting.[35] That said, this fast would be a great fast to start with considering the ease, safety, and proven results.

HOW TO KNOW IF YOU ARE MAXIMIZING AUTOPHAGY WHILE FASTING.

We must consider glucose and ketone measurements during extended fasting to determine your fasting and eating window, not to determine the length of your fast, but this time to determine if you are maximizing your autophagy and therefore your stem cell production.

As the fasting progresses, glucose should drop, and ketones should rise like the daily intermittent fast, but a more dramatic shift. Keep track carefully as the fast progresses. Ketone numbers should rise much higher than when in ketosis, with some people's ketones registering as high as 7.0–9.0 mmol/L. Glucose could drop as low as into the 30 range for some, which could be a major problem if the ketones are not rising to offset the energy low from glucose. I get emails from clients all the time saying my glucose is in the 40s or 50s, and is that ok? I then ask what their ketones are, and they will say 5.0–8.0. My response is to ask how they feel, and they most often say fine.

The key is the body is shifting over to fat-burning for its energy, so glucose drops, and the ketones rise as the fat burns.

There could be a day where ketone adaptation in the brain hasn't yet occurred, and you don't feel well yet, but give it a day, and the transition happens. My son Simon woke up Day 4 and said to me, "I thought you said I would feel better Day 4 when my ketones were up." He was 6.7 and still didn't feel well. I told him to wait, and his brain would adapt by the end of the day. Later that day he was out playing with bounding energy.

As for knowing if you are hitting maximum autophagy, according to keto and cancer researcher Professor Thomas Seyfried, it is when you hit what he calls the "Target Zone."[36] This zone is when your glucose and ketones hit a 1:1 ratio, meaning that if you divide your glucose number by 18, you get a European standard in mmol/L. You divide that number by the ketones which are in the same standard measurement of mmol/L, and it should be 1 or greater.[37]

For example, if your glucose is 80, you take 80 divided by 18 = 4.4 mmol/L. Then you take your ketones which are already in that standard and divide it by 4.4 so if they were 5.4 mmol/L, it would be 5.4 ketones divided by 4.4 glucose = 1.2 which is higher than one. This number would show that you exceeded the target zone and are maximizing autophagy. Hitting the target zone reflects the destruction of bad cells—if these numbers are showing up, the body is cleansing those bad cells and will replace them with stem cells to drive healing (Recycle/Renewal Principle). Cool, right?

Seyfried found this by watching tumors shrink or grow, so it was a fully correct way to look at autophagy. I was in a Mastermind in Orlando, Florida, with him, and when I heard him describe this, I applied it to my knowledge base of what I was doing and learning with my doctors. We then adopted it to find out it was an amazingly predictable tool.

HOW MY SON SIMON INSPIRED HUNDREDS TO FAST

When my son Simon was fourteen years old, he took his first fasting journey after being inspired by one of my clients whose eczema healed through a water fast. He saw my client's "before" picture and asked what was wrong with her. I explained it was a severe case of eczema like the small spots he had on his head. I then showed him the "after" picture, and Simon made a quick and very sure decision to fast.

He set out for a four to five-day fast I thought would end in half a day. To my surprise, he went far beyond five days. With no pressure from his mother or me, he found himself headlong into an eleven-day water fast. Before fasting, Simon was reaching for processed carbohydrates all day long to fuel his body, struggling with weight gain, some patches of eczema on his head, low energy, and sugar cravings.

SIMON'S FASTING STORY WILL ANSWER
MANY OF YOUR QUESTIONS

Simon's glucose dropped, and ketones increased by Day 2. Although ketones typically supply ample energy, Simon was not yet fat adapted on Day 2, and therefore was not using the ketones his body started producing. Some of his symptoms were nausea, lightheaded-ness, strong body odor, and welts around his knees. A white-coated tongue, tedious symptoms of illness, dizziness, and lack of energy typically accompany these first three days.

It is customary to start feeling better around Day 4 of a water fast. Simon felt better by the end of Day 4. He noted an increase in energy, and we saw his uplifted attitude, playing outside and improved sleeping habits. Forcing the body to use fat and ketones for fuel was a giant factor in improving Simon's sleep. How he was feeling was evidence that Simon's brain was using the ketones.

NOTE: If you do not feel better and make this transition into fat adaption by Day 4, circulating toxins and low electrolytes could be the reason.

Recall the three reasons you might not feel well and some solutions:

1. **Low electrolytes:** Add sea salt to your water to help maintain electrolytes. Taking magnesium may help some (I recommend magnesium malate or magnesium glycinate), or you may need to take a stronger, more balanced electrolyte-just find one without sugar.

2. **Not be fully fat adapted**: You may need to spend more time in the earlier steps or more variation in the diet weekly or monthly (see weeks 4 and 5).

3. **Still not fat adapted even following this protocol?** You may be struggling with some neurotoxicity. I recommend our "fasting trio" CytoDetox®, BIND, and Fastonic. However, some may have deep toxic issues and need one of our platinum doctors trained in Cellular Detox.

   - **Fastonic** down-regulates hydroxy free radicals. Free radicals cause inflammation and unwanted symptoms, especially during fasting.

   - **BIND** prevents the gut toxins from recirculating back into the body (auto-intoxication), which leads to many unwanted symptoms.

   - **CytoDetox®** helps support the body in the toxin elimination from the cells.

Before the fast, Simon's diet habits were very carb/sugar centered. Of all my children, Simon is the youngest and the one we were most hands off. He had the most food-addiction, and his first craving during the fast was for cheese. However, since breaking the fast, Simon attests to no longer having cravings or addictions. To date, all these symptoms left, and he eats amazingly. Fasting changed his life.

What controls the cravings and addictions is that ghrelin and leptin, hormones which affect the microbiome (gut bacteria), alter drastically during the fast and communicate to the hypothalamus to shut off hunger. Because of this, the body knows to avoid muscle. Frequently, when people try their hand at low-carb or low-calorie diets, the body doesn't avert from the muscle and taps into the muscle, and you become skinny fat; not a good look or a healthy one. With water fasts, innate intelligence recognizes muscle and protects it from being absorbed. Besides this, the body knows to go into autophagy, which we've discussed before, is the burning out of bad cells and fats.

Water fasting supplies a good chance to change your palate. For parents of vegetable haters, there is hope! A great breakthrough time was when

Simon (who previously had an aversion to vegetables of any kind), came off his fast, tried some broccoli, and enjoyed it. Also, we discovered his slight intolerance to dairy when he tried to delve back into cheese, unsurprising since conventional dairy can be a root issue to many chronic gut problems for individuals.

With ketones hitting 6.5 or greater and glucose ranging in the 40–50 range, Simon shed around fifteen pounds of weight. These are perfect target numbers for autophagy as he exceeded the "Target Zone." For a fourteen-year-old, the process has brought many spectators reciting that "if he can do it, I can do it." His fast has impacted hundreds if not thousands, to have the courage to fast.

MOST COMMON QUESTIONS ESPECIALLY WITH WATER FASTING

#1 QUESTION WE GET: WHICH WATER IS BEST?

This question is more important when water fasting but still a question that comes up during a partial fast or Fasting Mimicking Diet. For those who question what type of water is okay during a fast, distilled, sparkling, or filtered, here is an answer. It's beneficial to recall that we're not teasing the body with gullies of water, but rather depriving it of food sources to stimulate autophagy. It is worth checking in with your intention at this point because to reap the most benefits of true, deep, cellular healing, the body requires only plain, clean water.

Dedicate yourself to the process, without trying to "cheat" or get away with flavorings, additives, bubbles, or anything of the sort. Many people preach fasting with the use of such additives, and others include coffee, but, if you chose a water fast, do a true water fast: Water only. Apart from triggering your internal clock/metabolism, additives (including bubbly water) also trigger hunger response, which will make your fast more difficult. You are fasting for a purpose and can return to your preferred alternative waters once you complete the fast.

Fasting with tap water is out of the question because if your goal is to detox and heal your body, you do not want to be reintroducing pollutants into your body. Though blessed with abundant water free of parasites and bacteria, it comes at the expense of other chemicals. Chlorine alone is a powerful chemical that destroys gut bacteria just like antibiotics. Constituents such as lead, copper, and fluoride, which are neurotoxic chemicals that are not body-friendly, contaminate taps. Tap water can induce poor digestion, a weakened immune system, trigger autoimmunity, neurological disease, thyroid disorders, and skin diseases (like acne, psoriasis, and rosacea).

As far as filtered water goes, your best bet is a reverse osmosis whole home water filtration system. The reverse osmosis truly filters out all impurities and strips the water completely of minerals. Being mindful of this, occasionally add in a pinch of salt to your water to provide your body with some minerals and maintain electrolytes. When exploring the realm of water filters, note that many filters do not remove many (or any) pollutants found in tap water. Certain popular pitcher-style filters remove nothing but debris, and their aluminum filters cause an increase in the toxic load of the water. If you invest in a stand-alone 10.5 or pitcher filter, look for a five-gallon activated carbon gravity filter.

Distilled water is water that has been boiled into steam and condensed back into a liquid; basically, it is the water vapor. You can use distilled water for a water fast.

Spring water bottled in glass, or well water, are two excellent options for use during a water fast. These water sources are directly from nature and thus about as pure and natural as it gets, but you must know your sources. Not all spring waters are created equal. Buy it in stores (in glass bottles only) or use a spring water delivery service. You can always look at the testing that third parties do on different waters or have it tested yourself. If you are collecting it yourself, make sure your spring or well gets tested every couple of years to make sure there is no contamination by anything such as farm run-off.

Sparkling water is fine but can irritate the gut. My advice is to go easy on it.

A few words on adding sea salt:

These first few days can be difficult to get through. You are losing a lot of water, glycogen, and electrolytes, all of which can stimulate hunger allowing your body to burn more muscle than it would normally need to.[38] Adding sea salt to your water helps you to keep trace electrolytes, especially potassium, which helps protect your muscle. I recommend at least two round teaspoons of sea salt throughout the day. You may not want it in your water. Some people prefer to eat salt. Some people decide they don't want to take sea salt anymore.

Trace minerals or topical magnesium are also great alternatives to helping to keep minerals up during a fast. Electrolytes are your friend and will help to curb your appetite and hunger as well give you more energy. If you sip your water warm with a pinch of salt, it can also mimic sipping a warm broth, and be satiating. Listen to your body. It will tell you when to and if you should add a little salt to your water. With that said, here is question #2 for you.

#2 QUESTION WE GET: EXERCISE AND WATER FASTING, YES OR NO?

Can you partake in physical activity during a fast? Regarding fasting and movement, it's best to tread lightly. The best advice I can give is to rest during the fast and let the body focus on its healing. We fast to remove the stress of digesting and divert the energy to healing.

When we eat, the energy goes to digesting and takes away from heal-ing, and this is the same for exercise. We want our energy to go to healing mode, so now is the perfect time to take that recovery week and rest the body.

Exercising requires so much energy so quickly, and the body is tap-ping into muscle and may use gluconeogenesis (break down muscle for energy) to create glucose.39 Although the fast may not void you of energy (in fact, you may be amazed at the energy you feel), exer-cise can use vital energy need for healing. It's true that the healthier you are, the more you can exercise during a fast. I have tried some exercise with clients who have health challenges and found that most do worse the day after, so go easy here. Daily life is exempt, and simple tasks are fine for most to carry out. Water fasting is a time for cellular healing; conserve energy and let the body take care of itself.

Any stress to the body releases cortisol, which also increases glu-cose.40 You want to keep activity and emotional stress as well to a minimum. Rest is best!

With that said, there is a big jump in growth hormone on Day 5 of the fast.41 If you are going to exercise, this would be the day to try it and see how you do for the next fast.

QUESTION #3: CAN I DRINK MY COFFEE?

During any five-day extended fast, the answer is NO. Whether it's water, partial, or Fasting Mimicking Diet, the answer is still NO. Re-call that even during a daily intermittent fast, you must test to make sure your coffee is not raising glucose and breaking you out of au-tophagy. However, in an extended fast, there is no testing necessary because the answer is NO. Sorry, but we want to rely on the innate intelligence to do its healing without pushing the body in any direc-tion. Let the innate intelligence do the healing.

QUESTION #4: CAN I TAKE MY SUPPLEMENTS?

During a water fast, the only things allowed are electrolytes, and perhaps the Fasting Trio to minimize detox symptoms. Other than that, let the body do the healing.

During a partial fast or a ProLon *Fasting Mimicking Diet™*, you can add some of your favorite supplements, but this is a valuable time to give your body a break

THE FAST

I hope that you have a better sense of the "why and how" behind fasting, and that we've given you a clearer sense of where to start and what's best for you. This ancient healing strategy has changed many lives when no other tool worked. Sometimes the simplest and oldest proven strategies provide the most profound results.

With that said, let's partake in a five-day fast, which my wife Merily endearingly named "Fasting for a Purpose." Are you ready to bring your healing to a whole new level during Week 6? Ready for some "off the charts" autophagy going on? Ready to optimize your hormones? Let's do this! I set each day up with what you can expect to happen on that day, tips to help make the day easier, and some takeaways.

FIVE-DAY FAST: DAY ONE

NOTE: Continue medications but check with your doctor because you may need adjustment throughout the fast.

Start the practice of self-control with some penance; begin with fasting.

-Mahavira

The first day of your five-day fast has arrived. There may be many feelings surrounding this, such as fear of the unknown. Remember to determine your healing intentions and write them down. Focus on them and believe this will help you on your journey to true healing. Let's get this going!

Recommendations Before Starting

1. Journal your daily symptoms, feelings, emotions, thoughts, and breakthroughs.

2. Journal your intentions, physically, emotionally, and spiritually and pray over them daily — expect breakthroughs.

3. Expect God to move for you and others for whom you are fasting.

What to Expect on Day One

- It's normal for most to feel weak, tired, brain foggy, and hungry Days 1 and 2.

- Notice your tongue color throughout the fast. You may have significant white or yellowness in the tongue even after 24–48 hours. I've even seen black with some people, but that happens after many days. All of this will pass in time and is a normal reaction to detoxing. The tongue changes can occur on any day during these five days, and the colors can change. Include these changes in your journal, and you can compare them to other days of the fast, as well as later fasts.

- The first 2–3 days, you will experience a drop in glucose, but your body will make more ketones to supplement the energy loss. However, most of you will still feel weak and tired because you are not yet using the ketones efficiently. If you are more fat adapted (if you followed this program carefully before the fast, you should be pretty fat adapted), your ketones may even rise faster the first day, and you will use them sooner.[42] We want glucose to drop and ketones to rise, but since this is only Day 1, don't expect too much.

- If you are not yet fat adapted, you may feel the effects of low glucose the first couple of days - shakiness, "hangry," headaches, irritability, and nausea, to name a few. This situation will pass; give it time for your body to keto-adapt and start efficiently using the ketones. Rest, drink to thirst.

- Rashes are normal during any day of a fast and expect these anomalies and don't be intimidated by them. The body will get rid of toxins, and if these symptoms continue, you may need the supplements suggested for those who are having difficulty. However, start with some Epsom salt baths or a coffee enema and see if this relieves the symptoms.

- You may also experience some weird sensations any day during the fast. "Retracing" is where the body re-experiences and heals old illnesses or traumas that were incompletely healed in the past. As the fast progresses, this will happen more.

Keep in mind: Everyone heals at a different rate. Most of us are in a driving or growth mode, which is how we make cancer cells and age prematurely. The fasting process drives us into the opposite direction, into repair mode.[43]

Tips for Day One

- Mix sea salt in warm water, drink to thirst to help with nausea, curb the appetite, and calm the entire digestive system. Not everyone needs the sea salt, but in the first few days, it can help. If you are struggling with nausea, try it.

- Avoid supplements on a water-only fast. If you choose a water fast, it is water only and the meds you have cleared with your doctor. We don't want to push the body one way or another. Only if toxicity becomes a problem do we recommended three supplements that don't push the body but help the body get rid of the toxins.

- Avoid coffee and tea as well on a water-only fast. Coffee can make cortisol rise, which increases insulin and glucose, whereas water is neutral and allows the body to do what it needs to do (innate intelligence). We are resting the gut, resting our digestion, and forcing the body into a healing mode.

- Be careful with water temperature when showering, as too hot or too cold can push the body and raise cortisol. Take lukewarm showers and baths.

- Coffee enemas can help the first few days but are unnecessary. They may overstimulate some people, may help push things out for others.

- Don't over-complicate it. Drink water when you are thirsty. You don't need as much water as you think. You need not guzzle water all day long. Over-drinking can stress the kidneys. Listen to your body signals.

- Fasting is an art. During every fast, deeper healing occurs.

- If symptoms persist after Epsom salt baths or coffee enemas, consider CytoDetox®, BIND, and Fastonic.

- If symptoms are severe, contact your doctor.

Takeaways for Day One

It's normal to feel weak, brain foggy and be hungry Day 1. Your body is in a transition from glucose to fat for fuel for your body and ketones for the brain.

Always check in with your doctor before stopping any medication. You may still need some, such as diabetic and thyroid medications. These are okay to continue to take while fasting. Most people will find they need to take less of some medications. Always consult with your doctor before changing doses or stopping a medication.

FIVE-DAY FAST: DAY TWO

Everyone can perform magic; everyone can reach his goals if he is able to think if he is able to wait if he is able to fast.

- Hermann Hesse, Siddhartha

You hit Day 2, and your appetite might be all over the place. You will see food, and you will want food! All I can say is to hang in there on Day 2. By the end of the day, you're going to get a little low on energy. Your body is making ketones (if you measure your glucose and ketones, you will probably notice that your ketones are rising, and glucose is falling). Maybe your ketones are registering between 2.5, some of you 3.0, perhaps even higher. The issue is that you might not be using these ketones quite yet, as the body has not fully adjusted. If you have been following this protocol week by week, then hopefully you are already fully fat adapted and struggling less. It varies from person to person based upon your biochemistry.

What to Expect on Day Two

- Expect to feel hungrier and more irritable today, especially around the times you usually eat. There are physiological reasons for irritability; your glucose will be lower, and your brain is not happy because its energy supply is low. It can't use fat, and it's not adapting to only ketones yet.

- You may experience a lack of brain functioning and increased brain fog. Your brain loves ketones, but ketones are not high enough yet to be used efficiently. They will continue to rise, and you will feel better as you keto adapt; give it time.

- You may start lacking energy, especially if this is your first fast, or are having trouble in the earlier weeks getting into a ketogenic state.

Five Physiological Things That Will Happen on Day Two

Some major benefits play out on Day 2. Your body's innate intelligence is kicking into full gear, responding, and protecting. You may still feel poorly, I do not disregard this, but there are still some exciting accomplishments taking place.

- Cellular Autophagy: The body is getting rid of the defective stuff, specifically white blood cells that have been around too long (Recycle).[44]

- Rise in stem cells: Your body creates new cells such as white blood cells and gets rid of bad proteins in the muscle. Stem cells replace those tissues. Muscle fibers heal and adapt much faster (Renewal).[45]

- Reset DNA: We all have certain bad genes that are turned on. Fasting turns these off - obesity genes, allergies, and so forth.[46]

- Reset microbiome: There is a change in cravings, and a change of the ratio of good/bad bacteria, to help with losing weight and keeping it off.[47]

- Resets the gastrointestinal tract, and it begins to heal: Struggling with digestive issues? Resting digestion will give it the time it needs to begin healing.[48]

Tips for Day Two

- Continue to set your healing intentions; pray or meditate if you have spiritual beliefs as this helps tremendously during this first couple of rough days. Focus your prayer or meditation on the intentions you wrote.

- Continue to write more intentions for healing each day. Writing intentions down brings forth a birth to them.

- Distract yourself. This day is good to watch movies to help pass the time and keep you distracted. Another great tool is listening to podcasts or resources related to the benefits of fasting. They are extremely motivating and reassuring that the hardship is worth the effort. My friend Jeff goes to movies every day.

- Rest. Rest. Rest. Now is not the time to lift heavy weights or go for a run. Use this time to rest and heal. Conserve your energy. If you are doing too much, the body releases more cortisol, and this makes glucose goes up. Through rest, magic happens!

- Test glucose and ketones. The best time to test is the first thing in the morning, then do it again later in the day. You should see glucose trending down, and ketones trending up. Recall, a reading of above .5 ketones means you are in ketosis. All of you will be above that at this point but check to see if you are in the "Target Zone" for max autophagy. Many of you will already be there heading into super autophagy. However, your brain may not be using those ketones yet, so you may still feel poorly.

  NOTE: When glucose is high, you are not getting the full benefit of the ketones, so we want to see the glucose drop and ketones rise. The lower glucose and the higher the ketones, the more autophagy you will get. As the day goes on, you will see that transition occur.

- If you are still experiencing symptoms, try increasing your electrolytes.

- If symptoms are severe, this could be detox and CytoDetox®, BIND, and Fastonic may be a relief. See Day 1 suggestions like coffee enemas and Epsom salt baths.

Takeaways for Day Two

- It takes a great deal of cellular energy to digest food. When you eat a meal, the focus it takes for your innate intelligence to digest that meal is extreme. Take that digestion away from the equation, and you have a massive amount of focus and energy for healing. If you recall from the seven benefits of fasting, energy diversion is starting and will increase throughout the fast. When you simplify digestion and shift your energy to healing, magic happens.

- Gluconeogenesis may occur: Your body makes glucose from the muscle. It typically only happens for twenty hours and then shuts off to survive. The more you fast, the less this happens to where it does not happen for the experienced adapted faster.

- Ketones are rising, and glucose is falling. Low glucose = high ketones = more autophagy. Elevated ketones heal the brain, downregulate inflammation, and help the gut microbiome.

Please Note: The detoxing process induces the Herxheimer reaction, whereby the body feels worse before it feels better. This process can be extremely challenging for very neurotoxic people (Lyme disease, heavy metals, autoimmune conditions, cancer) who may need a coach throughout this process. These people may not feel better during the fast and would receive help from following my multi-therapeutic approach, with a coach.

FIVE-DAY FAST: DAY THREE

What to Expect on Day Three

- Your ketones will continue to rise on Day 3. Your brain loves ketones. Ketones fix the brain,[49] therefore, we use them for seizures[50] and neurodegenerative conditions[51] and dementia[52] and Parkinson's.[53] Ketones help to down-regulate cellular inflammation, heal the gut,[54] and reset your bad genes and turn on good genes.

- Hormone optimization: You get a growth hormone spike on Day 3. On Day 5, you will get the highest spike of growth hormone,[55] but the hormones will spike today. On Day 3, you get more sensitive to all your hormones,[56] and you may begin to feel better.

- You will start overcoming headaches, weakness, and shakiness. Woo- hoo! It's about time! The body starts ramping up stem cells and knocks down the overreaction of autoimmunity via autophagy.[57]

- You may have unexplained pains, meaning healing is occurring. For example, if you have an old knee injury, you may experience painful sensations in that knee. The body is going back through old injuries and trauma and healing them with its newly diverted energy.

- You may have increased energy and creativity; your body is no longer focusing on digesting food. It can divert the focus to other areas and direct its energy on brain focus and healing and can give you a whole new level of clarity you have not yet experienced.

- Hormonal changes may occur as the microbiome in your gut resets. Substantial changes are happening.

- You may feel some stomach and intestinal changes and upset. When we fast, we starve all bacteria, and this is usually self-limiting and part of the healing. However, we re-inoculate Day 6 with beneficial bacteria to take advantage of the drop in bacteria. Good and bad bacteria drop, but by re-inoculating with the good, we can overcome a severe dysbiosis of the gut.

- You may feel colder than usual. Why are you cold? Being cold is normal. Amazing things happen with the hormones. Certain hormone levels rise, and some may go down, but the cells become more sensitive to your hormones. Fasting lowers T3 thyroid hormone (innate intelligence playing out here) to spare your muscle and divert energy to more important things. So, we feel cold. The body knows what it is doing. It takes the energy need to keep us warm and prioritizes survival and healing. Although T3 lowers, the body is more sensitive to smaller amounts of the hormone. It's able to use the hormones available. The energy is going to healing, and the innate intelligence will divert energy from keeping the body warm to healing.[58]

Tips for Day Three

- If you are not feeling well, try the Fasting Trio.

- Sleeping in complete darkness can help you sleep.

- Turning off Wi-Fi at night can help sleep.

- Maybe it's time to turn up the heat and get more blankets.

Takeaways for Day Three

- Autophagy is in high gear. Bad cells are ripping away. Many of us have retracing symptoms, an old injury you now feel again. The body sends cytokines, these signaling molecules which are stirring the white blood cells into that area that stimulate stem cells, and that brings the healing.[59] Recycle/Renewal is a good thing. With every fast, I experience new retracing symptoms, and it reminds me of a past condition or injury.

- Most of us have too many bad bacteria, also known as dysbiosis. Bacteria gets reset, and we have a new microbiome starting Day 3.

- Hormone optimization: You experience a growth hormone rise on Day 3. Day 5, you get the highest spike of growth hormone. On Day 3, you get more sensitive to all your hormones, and you begin to feel better.

- Regarding bowel movements: Why are you not pooping? Because you are not eating! It's normal to not poop during a water fast. You may poop the first couple of days, but then you will probably stop. You may also have an odd mucous bowel movement during the fast, as part of a detox reaction. All of this is normal and expected. If you chose a partial fast or the FMD fast, you would go much less but still have small bowel movements.

FIVE-DAY FAST: DAY FOUR

What to Expect on Day Four—This should be the breakthrough day for most!

- Continued autophagy and new stem cell growth (Recycle/Renewal). Autophagy is at its high on Day 4.

- A continued drop in glucose and rise in ketones.

- Continued hormone optimization.

- Increased levels of energy and better brain functioning.

- The overall sense of well-being. Your brain is now using ketones efficiently. Your brain is keto-adapted. Congratulations!

- Decreased cravings, hunger, and irritability.

- You should be at max autophagy at this point. Recheck your target zone.

Tips for Day Four

- Increase prayer, meditation, or focusing on intentions to help keep cortisol levels down. If cortisol is down, so is glucose. We want to stay calm, relaxed, and full of positive intent during these last couple of days.

- Minimize stress (PHYSICAL AND EMOTIONAL) because cortisol increases glucose. Some ways to combat this: Don't overtrain; instead, increase your intentional prayer/meditation or focus towards healing.

- If symptoms are still getting worse and aren't the symptoms of not adapting that I have been describing, it is no doubt detox, and you should start the detox supplements or consider one of the Platinum doctors trained in cellular detox.

Takeaways for Day Four

Why is my glucose not dropping yet?

The bottom line why glucose is not dropping is that our mitochondria use glucose60 and fat for energy.[61] Toxins stored in the body damage the mitochondria.[62] The body is trying to find glucose in any way it can. It will use gluconeogenesis, the process by which the body breaks down muscle tissue to produce sugar. These people may not see remarkably high ketone levels and will see the glucose remain a little higher. Most Americans are stuck as glucose burners. However, through autophagy, the proteins used are typically cellular debris from damaged cells.[63] So we welcome the process and trust the body's innate intelligence to get rid of the bad cells since "bad cells don't adapt." So, with each fast and continued application of the principles you are learning in *Beyond Fasting*, you will progressively make better cells through the Recycle/Renewal Principle meaning that with each fast your numbers will keep improving. Healing takes time.

With that said, there is still the 800–pound gorilla in the room that can have a dramatic effect on your number and how you feel. Toxins affect the cell membrane (fatty membrane) and make their way into the cells and inflame the membrane and create inflammation. Toxins interfere with the hormone receptors needed to communicate with certain hormones, for example, thyroid hormone, insulin, and leptin. The hormones need to attach to hormone receptors to get their message into the cell, feel good, and burn fat for energy. When toxins come in and blunt these receptors, hormones cannot get their message to the cells.[64] Then you are not an efficient fat burner. When these toxins interfere with the mitochondrial membrane, that is when genuine issues occur with energy and ability to use fat.[65] Toxins are the **number one reason** we are stuck as glucose burners.

When you are stuck as a "sugar burner," even when you are not eating your body gives you cravings for carbohydrates, you can't resist because it wants to survive. When hormonally it cannot use fat for energy, it will break your muscle down to make sugar.[66] This is when you find high glucose numbers in the morning. It's normal to have slightly higher morning glucose known as the "dawn effect."

Cortisol and other hormones rise to dump some glucose and give you the energy to start your day, but high 90–100+ is too high. Most people are burning muscle to make glucose rather than burning fat, and therefore, they may wake up with a higher than normal glucose reading in the morning. Toxins disrupt the hormone's ability to burn fat.

How do you fix this?

More severe cases may need Health Centers of the Future Platinum Practitioners to coach you through cellular detox, especially if the Fasting Trio has not helped.

Multiple fasts = greater and greater efficiency and better and better numbers. It's the Metabolic Mitochondrial Fitness Principle (MMF).[67] Aim to embark on a five-day water fast every two to three months. Another choice is a partial fast or a Fasting Mimicking Diet every month for three to four months then try another water fast. With multiple fasts, glucose will drop faster, and ketones will rise more efficiently. You begin to feel better and better each time you fast because, in time, the mitochondria can use fat for energy. Multiple fasts change this gene (genes switch off and on with fasting) and fix the mitochondria via recycling the bad and making new more efficient ones.

Diet variation plays a key role here. Perhaps you started at the 5-1-1 and progressed to the 4-2-1 as outlined in this book, but many of you will benefit from a 3-3-1 with three fasting days and one feast day. Some may benefit from a 3-2-2 where you have two fasting days a week and two feast days. Everyone is different, but these variations using adaptation via hormone optimization with the feast/famine concept work.

WHAT'S GOING ON WITH MY SLEEP?

Sleep disturbances are common for the first few days. Yes, the first two days hunger pangs can keep you up, and all the changes taking place can disrupt your circadian rhythm and sleep cycle. However, the drop in glucose causes sleep problems, but once you become fat adapted, this should subside. I will say that as the fast goes on, I need less sleep and feel amazing. The "energy diversion principle" I describe is that the innate intelligence has so much more energy because of the energy not being used for digestion and assimilation of food. So much energy goes to this process from the gut to the cell that when it is not needed, the body diverts the energy to healing and there is still a surplus, especially if you are healthy.

Are you still having difficulty with sleep on Day 4? Sleep is one thing we look at for a diagnosis of neurotoxic illness. If you experience severe sleep disruption on Day 4, along with other symptoms such as severe fatigue, anxiety, and brain fog, most likely you are neurotoxic, and I recommended working with one of our trained practitioners to dig deeper. Disrupted sleep is also a sign your body is releasing toxins.[68] So hang in there!

With every subsequent fast, you get better, and more healing occurs. Your sleep may not be good on this one, but the next it will be better. Just as pains will come and go as the body is healing, so will sleep.

FIVE-DAY FAST: DAY FIVE

Yay! You made it to Day 5. Give yourself a big hug. Hopefully, you are feeling amazing at this point. There is no way you are quitting now! Here we will discuss how to break the fast tomorrow.

What to Expect for Day Five

- Stem cell production in high gear today. On Day 6 when you feed the stem cells, the body will heal and create new white blood cells for better immunity and other cells for what needs to be fixed![69]

- Ketones drop, glucose may slightly rise, but this is because you are using the ketones so efficiently for energy.[70]

- Massive growth hormone rise (goes up every day, but highest on Day

- 5) puts you in a healing mode that carries on beyond the fast.[71]

- Your body wants to survive, so it burns fat faster and more efficiently, to put [72] glycogen back in the liver.[73] Just in case it needs to run and save your life.

Tips for Day Five

- Consider continuing the fast with a partial fast starting tomorrow Day 6: 500–800 calories or move into a bone broth or bone broth with just oils (coconut oil, ghee) to continue the healing.

- This day is a terrific opportunity to transition back into a ketogenic diet for a few months after the two days of how to break the fast days.

- It is also an opportunity to transform your relationship with food. A fast will break your routine and offer you a clean slate to move forward with a more positive, healthy relationship with food. From addictions to overeating, under-eating, and cravings—examine aspects of your eating habits that are not serving your highest good and take this opportunity to let go of them.

- If you had an easy fast and are in good health, try working out on Day 5. Your high growth hormone advantage will give you huge benefits and could accelerate autophagy and stem cells on the refeed of Day 6.

Takeaways for Day Five

I mentioned that ketones might drop, and glucose may rise. You are oxidizing the ketones and using them for energy. When measuring beta- hydroxybutyrate, it's oxidized for energy.[74] Even normal activity like working and brain power/focus uses ketones for energy, which causes ketones to drop in the blood. However, you can evaluate the breath and ketones (the acetone from the ketones being oxidized and used) will be high.

WARNING: DO NOT RUIN YOUR FAST-Break the fast safely. Before you jump at the chance to throw a week's worth of nutrition down your throat, remember that you've just been in extensive, quiet healing: The digestive tract is still in rest mode. Your enzymes are low, and peristalsis (your gut's ability to move food through) is slow. A gentle transition is key to getting the best results from the fast and avoiding undermining efforts.

BEYOND FIVE DAYS: EXTENDED FASTING

What if I want to continue with the fast?

The first three days of a water fast are rough. However, after that, people tend to feel much better. What if you want to continue the fast beyond a five-day fast? Continuing beyond five days is what I refer to as "extended fasting." First, let's revisit some myths about fasting, as I'm sure you will get all kinds of unsolicited advice from naysayers while on your journey. You may hear things like, "It puts the body in starvation mode," and "It eats away at your muscles," and "It causes hypoglycemia," or "It's a yo-yo diet," or "Fasting causes hunger."

If my thirteen-year-old son Simon who was addicted to carbohydrates can tell you he is not hungry anymore after Day 3 (and feels good), there goes that hunger myth. Regarding starvation? Fasting puts the body into prevention mode. It prevents starvation from happening by preserving the muscle via hormone optimization and uses fat and bad cells for energy. These longer fasts will result in continued autophagy, thus increased stem cell production and cellular healing and may benefit some.[75] I will say that unless you are very overweight, I prefer multiple fasts for safety. A trained doctor should always supervise longer fasts.

What are some concerns I have with extending fasts beyond five days?

- If you have never embarked on a fast before, I do not recommend trying to do an extended fast without supervision. We have trained Platinum practitioners experienced in this program.

- You must fast for at least four days (sometimes longer) to get that benefit of becoming fat adapted, so do give it at least that long. Many people decide to go longer after they set a short goal of four days.

- If you are an inexperienced faster wanting to fast longer than four to five days, I recommend doing so with supervision from one of us trained in this program. I'm training doctors around the country for this purpose. Fasting is a part of what we do, along with true cellular detox and these ancient healing strategies and is what I call a *Multi- Therapeutic Approach* to healing. If you are sick or have never fasted, it is important to collaborate with a trained practitioner when undertaking an extended fast.

- Electrolytes are a concern for some and cause some severe complications. Long fasts require blood tests to watch potassium and sodium levels, which can drop with people who have certain health challenges.

- If you are on medication, check with your doctor because adjustments will be needed, especially on longer fasts. You will need to watch blood work for medication changes.

WHAT ARE SOME SIGNS YOU MAY NEED TO BREAK THE FAST ESPECIALLY IF ON A LONGER FAST BEYOND FIVE DAYS?

Tongue turns back to pink? Time to stop. This is truer on longer fast where the tongue turns nasty color, then all of sudden turns back to pink.

Hunger returns? Time to stop. Again more reliable on longer fast.

If you stop losing weight for one or two days? Time to stop. Longer fast only.

Extreme weakness or fatigue. SHOULD I FAST A FEW DAYS LONGER?

Under the supervision of a trained doctor, seven to eight days of fasting may improve benefits for some people. If you are feeling good during the fast, but numbers are still not great? Give it a couple more days. If you start feeling good on Day 5, give it another day.

Are you extending much longer than that? Do so under doctor supervision. **I recommend several five-day fasts to get the best improvement.** With each later fast more autophagy takes place, new stem cells form, and the body continues to heal exponentially.

DR. DERRICK DEMPSEY'S AND DR. DON CLUM'S
EXTENDED FASTING STORIES

I had the pleasure of having Dr. Derrick Dempsey on my *Cellular Healing TV* podcast.[76] Dr. Dempsey water fasted for twenty-two days, which he claims helped him tremendously with many of his health issues. Dr. Dempsey grew up with a pastor as his father. The ideology he experienced behind fasting was not if you fast; it was when you fast. The biblical ties to fasting are a huge gauge for many of us, including myself. The second "why" for fasting stemmed from his responsibility to family.

Dr. Dempsey's original plan was to complete a five-day water fast. However, his fast evolved into twenty-two days of fasting. Having experienced fasting with whey water and broth previously, he prepared for the task which brings us to the first concept in coaching—mental preparation. By Days 2 and 3, despite the longing for meals, Dr. Dempsey powered through. The switch, a sort of mindset alteration, occurred between Days 4 and 6, where he developed a slight aversion to food and his mental clarity recharged. "You're fine with water," he told himself. "Just keep going."

As his fasting progressed, Dr. Dempsey noticed some erratic changes in his mental ability. As a youth, bludgeoned down by four head traumas and never feeling recovered fully, he initially noted that his mental clarity skyrocketed. Like many of us, he previously would have to read and reread things several times over to get the gist. With fasting, however, Dr. Dempsey found this just was not the case. His acuity soared. Such is the case with brain fog.

A colleague of mine, Dr. Clum, beat out Dr. Dempsey's record, with a thirty-day water fast!

Like Dr. Dempsey, Dr. Clum, whom I also interviewed on *Cellular Healing TV*,[77] had not previously planned on the prolonged fast. What started as three days moved swiftly to five, and then to ten, and continued.

This fast wasn't Dr. Clum's first experience. He recounts instances with moles and lesions, non-biopsied but diagnosed skin cancers, which formed on his neck and back. These diagnoses inspired actions like juicing, fasting, which helped the lesions and moles to fight their way off his body within six months. Dr. Clum admits to the struggles of powering through but vocalizes his energy, positivity, and strength that levied in return during his fasts.

CAMILLE RECOUNTS LISTENING TO HER BODY DURING AN EXTENDED FAST

"When I embarked on my very first water fast, with no earlier fasting experience, I had the intention of completing seven days. The first six days were extremely low energy, and I spent most of the time in bed, relaxing, resting, and writing. I am an active person and rarely take a day off from the gym. My agenda is always packed, I am pushing myself to the limit and then some. Resting for me throughout the fast was difficult mentally because of my nature, but I knew it would help the deep cellular healing that was going on inside. On Day 7, I woke up full of energy as if I had been eating the whole week. With energy and strength completely restored, I was so tempted to keep fasting, but a bigger part of me knew that this is my nature; to take a good thing and push it to the point when it is no longer best. In the past, I would always overtrain (to the point of near adrenal exhaustion) and over-caffeinated myself.

Today, I have taken a step back and addressed my health much more holistically, understanding that balance is the foundation of a thriving body and that sometimes less truly is more. Despite having a strong urge to continue for ten or even fifteen days, I broke my fast at 170 hours (seven full days) as I had intended. Given my nature, this was a much greater sign of strength to stop than it would have been to continue onwards. Having completed the seven days without overdoing it, I have since incorporated extended water fasting into my lifestyle more regularly instead of pushing myself to the extreme any one time."

I wanted to include Camille's story because I have many people who have health challenges and who want to fast longer, for a feeling of victory or conquering, and maybe they even felt a little better. However, once again, what I have found is that multiple short fasts can be better for those more metabolically challenged. Often, my advice is: Instead of fasting on with water only, move onto a partial fast for another five days or so.

For anything related to health, many people tend to get wrapped up in extremes, and this is one of the main reasons healthy habits may not be sustainable, overall. Although many people have problems with overeating and too much exercise, a newly emerging problem is too much exercise and too much calorie deprivation. For fasting, listen to your body and trust in its wisdom. After you complete the five days, it may be tempting to continue onwards, but I urge you to tune into the intention and the place from where this temptation is coming.

I FEELING BETTER WHY AM I NOW SUDDENLY FEELING WORSE?

As you are fasting, the body is going through healing and releasing toxins.[78] If you go through periods of poor energy, headaches, flu symptoms, you may be experiencing some detox reactions because of bad bacteria, viruses, molds, toxins. You may not be healed metabolically yet. You may have a toxic build-up in your cells, and it can take several fasts to feel significant improvements. With major cellular toxicity, it may take multiple fasts, working with a trained practitioner, and my multi-therapeutic approach to healing.[79]

You've gotten rid of all these bad cells, and your body is making all these new stem cells. Week 7 is up next, refeeding, which may be the most important part, as there is a right way and a wrong way to refeed after fasting.

THE REFEED

**WARNING: DO NOT RUIN YOUR FAST AND HARD WORK.
READ THIS CAREFULLY!**

Congratulations, you made it to Week 7, and you earned it! This week is especially important; I can't stress this enough. We've "cleared the house" through a great deal of autophagy last week, and we've lowered our gut bacteria down, and this is a good thing because we want to fix gut problems such as dysbiosis, and reinoculate our gut with healthy bacteria. The stem cells are rising, and now they need to be fed. This week you will learn exactly how to feed them, and what to feed them.[1]

REBUILD AND REPOPULATE

Although the hardest part of the fast is behind you, the next three days are crucial in terms of the overall success of the fast. Your body is very fragile following an extended water fast; the autophagy processes your body underwent has left your gut and stomach as somewhat of a blank canvas. Think of your body as that of a newborn baby: You want to ease back into eating solids and harder-to-digest foods. You have starved the harmful bacteria out but also much of the good, so it is imperative to reintroduce probiotic rich, easy-to-digest foods to repopulate your gut and build back a healthy and stronger-than-ever stomach lining.

I've had clients who look at refeeding as devouring chocolate cake or eating a huge steak and believe me, they blow it. Let me explain why this is not a good idea and may sabotage all your efforts. What happens during the fast are your enzymes and bacteria lower down. If you throw a ton of food in there, you won't be able to digest it all effectively. Therefore, we need to go "low and slow" introducing food. We need to inoculate the gut with beneficial bacteria and enzymes.[2]

Recall the partial fast we discussed as a possibility for Week 6? The partial fast is also a way to break out of a fast. Keep the calories low (500–1000) for two to three days, sticking with basic and easy-to-digest foods. After three days, go back to your normal caloric eating. For me, this means eating in that intermittent fasting window. My window is typically four hours, but you stick with whatever window you found works best for you during the intermittent fasting week.

The key is keeping calories low, in that partial fast zone, because your enzymes are low. The last thing we want to do is throw a bunch of difficult- to-digest proteins in the mix. So, we will not consume any meat or grains yet. Soft-cooked vegetables are your friends for the first couple of days post fast. Raw vegetables may be too much on Day 1 post-fast, even raw salad. Steamed and blended vegetables are best. Fermented vegetables, like kimchi and sauerkraut, are great. You can find these in the refrigerated section of most grocery stores. These can help replace the good gut bacteria starved down during the fast.[3] Oils are good but keep it light on those first days. You can also try cultured cottage cheese, which has bacteria and enzymes.

What about dairy? If you tolerate dairy, you can add in some good grass- fed, preferably raw, fermented dairy, fermented full-fat yogurt, and kefir. These can help to feed that beneficial bacteria again, and all are soft.

What are my favorite "breaking the fast" foods? I like avocado with a little olive oil, salt, and pepper on it. I also really enjoy cultured cottage cheese. I love that on avocado. These are just some ideas, and we have a little meal plan for you with more ideas. My goal is to show you it's quite easy to break a fast, but I also want to be sure you do so without overeating so your body can manage it.

On Day 2, some of you can start slowly adding some salads (go easy), but I feel it's best to hold off on most raw vegetables and meat until Day 3. Eggs are a terrific addition for Day 2 because they're easier to digest than most meats.

Come Day 3, you can eat all the same foods you ate on Days 1 and 2, but this is the better day to eat more of the raw foods, like vegetables and salads. This day is where many people get tempted and break. The temptation will be a big meal. However, if you go low and slow, you will be grateful.

On Day 3, we're back to following the ketogenic diet, eating two meals per day within that eating window. Pick back up with the diet variation strategy 4-2-1. If you stick to these strategies you learned, your health and healing will keep going to the next level. I am healthy now and still practice these principles.

IMPORTANT NOTE: *The feeding fires up the new stem cells that are just waiting to do their job, and when we start this refeeding correctly (as I'm telling you), the stem cells will go to the places that need healing.*[4]

Remember that digestion starts in the mouth: Chew your food properly to ensure you absorb the most out of your food and ease the digestive burden on your stomach and gut.

Your digestive enzymes will be sluggish after the fast. Therefore, we want to go low and slow with easy-to-digest foods. Pay attention to calories, for you don't want to consume too much too fast. Once you are back to eating a regular whole foods diet, continue onwards with intermittent fasting to continue reaping the benefits of moving forward.

SAMPLE DIET: DAILY BREAKDOWN

Day One (Women: 500–800 calories/Men: 800–1000 calories)

- Bone Broth
- Soft-cooked vegetables (preferably cooked in the broth)
- 100% vegetable juice (ideally heavily or entirely green juice; many vegetables like beetroot and carrot are high sugar content, particularly when juiced)
- Berries and low glycemic fruit
- Avocado
- Sauerkraut (small quantities)
- High quality (grass-fed/organic) unpasteurized cottage cheese (raw), coconut milk kefir yogurt, raw milk, homemade coconut yogurt, and colostrum powder
- Probiotics
- Grass-fed ghee
- Coconut oil
- Olive oil

Day Two (Women: 800–1000 calories/Men: 1000–1200 calories)

- Same as Day 1 + organic pasture-raised eggs (if you tolerate eggs)

Day Three (Normal diet)

- Same as Day 2 + reintroduce organic pasture-raised meat, and all vegetables (cooked or raw), all fruits, nuts, seeds, supplements

ESTABLISHING A HEALTHY RELATIONSHIP WITH FOOD

Note that moving forward from Day 3, a "regular" diet does not mean the standard American diet. If you have struggled with food and diet in the past, this is an opportunity to develop a healthy relationship with food and your body. I highly encourage intermittent fasting moving forward and nourishing your body with real (preferably organic) food. Envision the nutrient-dense diet and lifestyle you would like to gift to your body and approach the transformation from a place of love. You've put in all this challenging work in the name of health, and this journey does not stop as soon as your fast finishes. If you plan on reintroducing unhealthy foods, I suggest giving your body at least four to six weeks with no junk to maximize your stem cell production and other post-fast health benefits.

Everybody has an individual relationship with food, so tune into what your body may or may not want from the suggestions above. Sauerkraut is an example of a food that might be too overwhelming for certain individuals to reintroduce on Day 1. You are your own best compass for what your body needs, so be mindful of that.

The weeks following a water fast also offer you the opportunity to explore food intolerances you may or may not have known you had. For some people, a fast will "reset" their body's ability to metabolize eggs, but for others, eggs will trigger a negative immune response. Be mindful when reintroducing food products that are common allergens. These foods include eggs, milk/dairy, peanuts, and other tree nuts (walnuts, almonds, pine nuts, brazil nuts), soy, wheat, and other glutinous grains, fish, shellfish, and nightshade plants (like eggplant, peppers, and tomatoes). Going straight back to a regular meal size will place an enormous digestive burden on your body, so take it slow.

DIGESTION

"You are what you eat" has without a doubt, been replaced with the notion that "you are what you digest." As you can see, the days following the fast are heavily rooted in building back your body's resilience and microbiome, to ensure you have a strong and thriving digestive system. Your gut health impacts everything from the way you think (gut-brain axis) to the health of your skin, your body's ability to fight off germs and infections, and so much more. I must emphasize the importance of your gut as the processing plant that turns food into nutrients and acts as the gatekeeper that lets these nutrients enter the body and nourish your cells. Leaky gut or malabsorption of food—which are becoming the norm in our modern times—is at the root of fueling a wide range of disease. Here are a few tips to perfect your digestion moving forward:

1. Digestion starts in the mouth: The active enzymes in your saliva break down food before it ever leaves your mouth. Slow down and eat mindfully. Chewing your food is integral to breaking it down into absorbable nutrients, and studies show that a mindful eating practice also helps with bloating and indigestion (CITE). Try to avoid electronic distractions while eating; be present with your food and anyone with whom you are eating.

2. Celery juice is a fantastic way to increase the body's endogenous production of hydrochloric acid (HCL or stomach acid), which is the next step in your digestive process after you properly chew your food. Drinking eight to sixteen ounces of fresh (preferably organic) celery juice first thing in the morning will boost your digestive strength throughout the day. Other digestive boosting morning tonics include lemon juice, and apple cider vinegar, both of which you should dilute in water.

3. There are many supplements you can introduce into your daily routine to give you added support in terms of digestion. These include digestive bitters, digestive enzymes, and an HCL+ pepsin combo.

WHAT DO I DO AFTER THE REFEED?
HERE IS HOW I LIVE MY LIFE

Start smaller; do a partial fast afterward. Consume fewer carbs, fewer calories as described. Go slower and simpler. Each fast after this will get easier.

You learned that during a fast, you might experience pain from past injuries, like knee pain or neck pain from an injury that occurred years ago. The pain you are experiencing is the autophagy and energy divergence working and may occur after the fast as well because we're refeeding the stem cells, and they are going to the site of the injury to help with continued healing.[5]

Therefore, it's important to break the fast correctly. Breaking the fast is not the finish line here! Often people heal increasingly through later fasts. With every fast, I felt healing from the rise in stem cells and autophagy, and experienced healing in various parts of my body each time.

Metabolically, we get more efficient and flexible with each fast. Many people tell me that by their second or third fast, they were in ketosis "just like that." For those of you who struggle to get into ketosis, notice the difference with each new fast. You will become more of what I refer to as "metabolically flexible." I am at a point now where I go in and out of ketosis easily. What this means is that if I've been out of ketosis for a few months, I can quickly get back into it because I fast weekly. I still do the 5-1-1 or the 4-2-1 variation I taught you. I even mix it up with 3-2-2.

We know the Hunza as the longest living, healthiest people on the planet. Many believed their longevity is because of *what* they eat. However, we now know it's *how* they eat—seasonally. In the summer, they are primarily vegetarian. In the wintertime, they go into full-blown ketosis. However, the key to their longevity is the spring. Every spring, they fast, and it's still a cultural principle. They have a name for it—"starving spring." I continue this tradition myself and fast every spring. I also like to fast in January, to bring me back into ketosis after the holidays. I'm a big believer in varying our diet seasonally, as this served ancient cultures well.

You have worked hard to become fat adapted with ketosis. Please keep it going for another few months and then vary your diet seasonally by cycling in a healthy higher-carbohydrate diet. My *Cellular Healing Diet* is an excellent example since by most standards, I would consider it to be low carbohydrate. However, compared to ketosis, it would still be a step toward higher carbs. Recall from the chapter on diet variation; the key is forcing the body to adapt to the dietary change and receiving help from the hormone optimization that occurs which is at the heart of Metabolic Mitochondrial Fitness (MMF). The more your diet changes and shifts, the stronger your cells and mitochondria become, and the more fat adapted and the more energy you produce via your body fat. Bad cells do not adapt, but good cells get stronger.

It's so tempting to stay on a diet you feel is working for you. However, I promise you, as pointed out by the science and years of experience, that you will gain greater benefit from the seasonal variation. With that said, weekly and seasonal variation should continue. You have all the tools you need in this book.

You are not at the finish line; this is just the beginning for most of you. With every fast,[6] you will become more metabolically flexible,[7] you will have a rise in stem cells, healing,[8] and more autophagy.[9] For the average person, you can partake in one to two fasts a year and still reap the benefit. We have heard that one fast a year decreases cancer by 95%. However, if you are more metabolically challenged, more frequent fasting throughout the year will help. For example, do one fast quarterly, and some may benefit monthly, but be sure to interchange this with water fasting and partial fasting or a Fasting Mimicking Diet.

HOW DO I CONTINUE AFTER THE REFEED ESPECIALLY WITH AUTOIMMUNITY ALLERGIES FOOD SENSITIVITIES, AND METABOLIC ISSUES?

Autoimmunity, allergies, and food sensitivities have all become an epidemic. Most of us are undiagnosed and just not feeling well and not sure why. Multiple fasting is the answer. We have seen this clinically, and solid science backs it. In autoimmunity, we have too many immune cells living too long, thus becoming over-reactive and hypersensitive which in turns drives the immune system to either attacking itself or overreacting to something as simple as pollen or a protein from food. What we have seen with multiple fasts is that each fast gets rid of these old cells via autophagy and creates new, less reactive, naïve stem cells.

Once your body has become more metabolically flexible and able to shift in and out of ketosis, you can make dietary shifts not only seasonally but also weekly. For example, my wife and I can be in ketosis for a week or two, because we now can get into ketosis in one day, and then move back out for a week or two. Varying the diet is the key.

People spend big money to have stem cells injected. We call this program *Beyond Fasting* because I have taught you how to raise your stem cells and turn back aging, a system that will forever change you. Congratulations on taking this journey. Keep connected on my Facebook fasting group, with even more information and support. Please keep reading to learn about some of my favorite post-fast healing strategies.

CELLULAR DETOX: A SOLUTION TO WHY YOU STRUGGLE TO FAT ADAPT AND DO NOT FEEL WELL

I have talked a lot about neurotoxin effect on your ability to fat adapt, and as a reason you may not be feeling well. Therefore, I want to expand on the three products in the Fasting Trio and the Cellular Detox used by myself and the Platinum Practitioners.

THE FASTING TRIO: CYTODETOX®, BIND, AND FASTONIC

Cellular toxicity may be why you are not fat adapted and may not feel well during a fast. We often use these three products during a fast, and even during ketosis, to mitigate many of the symptoms associated with these transitions. These may be enough for many of you. However, if you are highly toxic or have more complicated health conditions, they will not be. Therefore, you may need a more in-depth cellular detox. I've trained Platinum practitioners around the country in the protocols of this book and my thorough True Cellular Detox process.

I rarely recommend supplements during a water fast, as I'm not eager to push the body one way or another. I like to rely solely on the innate intelligence of the body. However, these three supplements do not push the body left or right. CytoDetox® is a particle, not an herb or a vitamin. BIND stays in the gut and therefore doesn't affect you systemically, and

Fastonic is a hydrogen molecule (not an oxidant or an antioxidant). It's called a redox molecule, and all three work with your body's innate intelligence.

CYTODETOX®

Safe cell detoxification of chemicals and heavy metals is vitally important if you want to achieve healthy cellular function. Years ago, I lost my health and almost my life to heavy metal toxicity. I needed to find a substance powerful enough to support my body to detoxify mercury and usher it out of my sick body. However, true heavy metal binders like a clean clinoptilolite zeolite were far and few between in the search.

Supposed natural heavy metal chelators, such as cilantro and chlorella, proved to be too weak to bind to the heavy metals, allowing these toxins to re- circulate back into the fatty tissue and cells of my body. These natural binders may show some binding ability in a glass beaker or lab setting. However, once in the gut, the microbial activity typically eliminates and alters these plant-based structures, making them unable to truly bind toxins. Therefore, these natural plant chelators are not true binders.

Dimercaptosuccinic acid or DMSA is a true binder, and I used it successfully back when I was sick. However, accessing a decent quality DMSA has become a challenging task because of recent regulations. When we realized we no longer had easy access to DMSA, I faced some challenges. I became concerned about my sick clients. When you are detoxing heavy metals, you MUST have a true binder that can support the body's natural ability to detoxify. We did not have a good option for them.

My wife said, "You need to pray about this." One week later, I received a call about the active ingredient now in CytoDetox®, which was a new form of zeolite that turned out to be the answer to our prayers. I was skeptical until I learned more about this new structure. We tested it with both our laboratories and our large health practitioner network. The results are in—it was clean and effective.

One of the biggest problems with these types of products is that they are such good binders that they bind and hold on to toxins, such as lead and arsenic. We also tested almost every product on the market containing these binding particles, and all of them have these contaminants and more. We now have a patented process to clean the particles, and I can say CytoDetox® is the only clean product on the market.

As far as testing effectiveness, one problem was the size of the particles and keeping its ability to bind. With standard zeolites on the market, their particle structures are large and typically will not cross the gut unless broken down into smaller particles. What we found is that the smaller particles in many of the products lost their ability to bind. Therefore, we had to find a way to bring active binding particles across the gut without losing the binding ability. Liposome technology was the answer.

When using real binders like CytoDetox, you move many toxins from the cell out of the body and can create redistribution. My vision was to make the product even more effective with fewer symptoms. Smaller particles penetrate the cell, but we also needed to support larger particles that stay outside the cell to prevent toxins from redistributing. We experienced great success as the new CytoDetox has many small particles that can cross into the cell and its membranes where the toxins live, and larger particles stay outside of the cell to make sure all the toxins exit the body.

For over three years now, our practitioner network has used CytoDetox® for cell detoxification support with amazing analytical test results and health testimonials. Now, with the new and improved CytoDetox® and the CytoDetox® Plus, we expect even more amazing results, testimonies, and gratitude to pour into our in-boxes.

When looking at upstream toxins, such as heavy metals and environmental chemicals embedded in most of our organs, glands, cells, and brain tissue, we know it is of utmost importance to deal with high toxicity promptly and safely. Unfortunately, you can't just do a liver or kidney cleanse once a year and believe that it thoroughly cleanses you. It is impossible to single out an organ and limit cell detoxification to one part of the body. Even if we could select toxins from the liver one at a time, we could only remove an estimated 2% or 3% of the toxic load.

Toxins pass through the liver for removal but often end up deposited in fatty tissue and other body tissues, including the brain. What we can do is take CytoDetox® to support the body's natural ability to pass toxins through the liver, and usher them out of the system for complete cell detoxification support. CytoDetox® does not limit itself to supporting the removal of heavy metals such as mercury, lead, cadmium, and arsenic. CytoDetox® can fully support the body for a wide variety of positively charged toxic exposures.

BIND

The BIND (Toxin Elimination) formula provides a specialized form of activated charcoal and powerful humates (humic and fulvic acids) along with key botanicals that effectively bind toxins and prevent retoxification. BIND serves as a master drainage formula that attracts toxins, binds them, so they don't reabsorb, and escorts them out of the body. Most toxins, especially during fasting, are brought to the liver to be processed and hopefully excreted. Many of the toxins bind up to bile.

Bile is a fatty substance used to break fat down in the intestines but because it is fatty, attracts the toxins and hold them in a complex known as hepatic biliary sludge. It is what it sounds like—toxic liver sludge. The problem is that when you use your bile to digest fat, it brings the toxins in this complex with it. The bigger problem is that your body is designed to reabsorb the bile back to the liver. Therefore, it brings the toxic bile complex (hepatic biliary sludge) with it and creates what we call auto- intoxication. BIND sits in the gut like a catcher's mitt and pulls the toxins out of the gut and prevents the autointoxication that manages so many of the unwanted symptoms during a fast or detoxification.

Benefits of BIND:

- Contains super-activated charcoal.

- Absorbs up to 300 times its weight in toxins.

- Cascara Sagrada brings water into the intestines.

- Apple and flax provide beneficial fiber.

- Probiotics added to support leaky gut.

- Alkaline has a negative ion charge that electromagnetically binds with positively charged toxins (heavy metals).

- Sweetens the intestines (absorbs gases that the liver would otherwise have to handle) and prevents flatus.

- Absorbs pathogens (virus, bacteria, parasites, mycoplasma) and their metabolic wastes.

- Does not interfere with nutrient absorption or intestinal function.

- Favorably impacts cholesterol via binding the bile complex.

- Helps to prevent bloating.

- Daily use can lower the body's toxic exposure by 60%.

- Helps trap pesticides, herbicides, and plastics from consumed non- organic foods.

- Ultimate quality, super activated, highest binding ability.

- Fulvic acid transports minerals throughout the body and supports cellular fluidity.

- Humic acid smothers viruses and prevents their attachment to cell membranes.

- Binds bio-toxins (Candida, molds) in the intestines, prevents re-absorption.

- Humates supply over seventy plant-source trace minerals.

- Promote healthy enzyme reactions.

FASTONIC

Molecular hydrogen H2, the smallest and most bioavailable molecule in the Universe, is formed when two hydrogen atoms combine and provide the body with great benefit. Inflammation causes many of the unwanted symptoms during fasting, but we don't want to take antioxidants during a fast, as they can neutralize key oxidants that drive autophagy and healing in your immune system. However, too much inflammation, especially in those with toxic issues and health challenges, can drive unwanted symptoms.

The redox mechanism in Fastonic, using hydrogen molecular technology, finds a perfect balance of working with and not against the innate intelligence. This innovative technology and understanding of "redox" have changed the way we think of antioxidants and their usage. Too much lowers immunity and too little can drive inflammation and its destruction. We have learned we can't figure it out, and the safest, most effective therapy is to give redox signaling molecules, and let the body's wisdom figure it out. Fastonic enters the new frontier of anti-aging.

We know the cellular, molecular hydrogen in Fastonic will:

- Promote a healthy balance of oxidative stress, neutralizing only the most harmful free radical into water.

- Support glucose homeostasis.

- Promote healthy function of inflammation system.

- Help stabilize cholesterol levels.

- Stimulate energy metabolism to prevent age-related weight gain.

- Support cognitive function, increasing mental clarity, and focus.

- Increase the rate of healing from soft tissue injuries.

- Reduce fatigue experienced during and after exercise.

- Improve skin health and appearance.

- Be a source of highly bioavailable magnesium.

TRUE CELLULAR DETOX (TCD)

I've stated repeatedly that many of you do not feel well during the fast even on Day 4 or 5 or are struggling to become fat adapted during ketosis, and this is most often because of cellular toxicity. Toxins disrupt the cells' natural detox pathways, which may lead to other cellular function problems such as the cells' ability to use fat in the mitochondria for energy. The Metabolic Mitochondrial Fitness (MMF) that we use through diet variation is a highly effective strategy to make the mitochondria stronger and more efficient. Recall that bad cells do not adapt. Therefore, they either get stronger or die, and we create new, more efficient cells (via stem cells). However, with some people, because of toxins, these strategies are not enough without True Cellular Detox.

Most detoxes you find in practitioners' offices, and health food stores are down-stream, where the real problem lies. The fact is that cells have natural detox pathways to remove not only the toxins we are exposed to but also the endogenous toxins made in the cell when the cell produces energy. These toxins are normal parts of cellular energy and metabolism. However, when the cells' detox pathways start shutting down, toxins will accumulate in the cell. This situation leaves us in a state of cellular dysfunction, and possibly sickness and disease. Most often, this is why we don't feel well. We must fix the cell to get well, and in this case, detoxify the cell to get well.

True Cellular Detox (TCD) is a process I learned and created through my health challenges, and those of whom I coach back to health and works by improving cellular function, so the body can detox and heal itself. This approach incorporates my 5Rs of True Cellular Detox and Healing, which has become a road map for not just fixing the cell, but also for detoxification.

Three components and three phases make up real detox.

The Five R's

1. Remove the source.
2. Regenerate the cell membrane.
3. Restore cellular energy.
4. Reduce cellular inflammation.
5. Re-establish methylation.

THE THREE COMPONENTS THAT MAKE UP REAL DETOX

1. Real detox occurs in the cell. You must upregulate cell function, not just deal downstream with colon and liver cleanses.

2. We must open the downstream detox pathways, and address the liver, kidneys, lymph, and the gut as part of the process to help in the complete removal of the toxins from the body. Otherwise, redistribution of the toxins will create unwanted symptoms, and potentially you become worse, not better.

3. We must use real binders. Real binders are critical to prevent toxins from redistributing and recirculating back into other parts of the body, such as the brain. Therefore, most detox products not only fail but can also be dangerous. Most products contain weak binders that do not bind the most dangerous types of toxins (such as heavy metals) strongly enough to bring them entirely out of the body. I've authored several articles on this on my website called, "When Detox is Dangerous."

TCD works to repair the natural detox pathways of the cell upstream, while keeping the downstream detox pathways open (lymph, liver, kidneys, and gut), and includes true binders to aid in the removal of toxins.

THE THREE PHASES TO TRUE CELLULAR DETOX

First, there is a one to two months "prep phase" for detox pathways at the cell and downstream where the goal is to start supporting the cell function (via the 5Rs) and not push to the point of detox until the pathways strengthen. Even after the prep phase, it is important to note that the cellular pathways and the downstream pathways need support throughout every phase of the process. After the one to two months of the prep phase, we move into a "body phase" that typically lasts three to four months, and finally the most crucial phase of all, the "brain phase."

Some typical types of cleanses, such as colon cleanses or coffee enemas can be helpful in the later phases of detox (body phase and brain phase) to keep the toxins moving out of the body and not backing up, causing unwanted symptoms. A simple cleanse like this can be useful before or during TCD, but if you end there, you will never make it to where the actual problem exists.

The brain phase is where the magic happens. Eventually, applying this process to the brain using fat-soluble detox agents with the CytoDetox (that not only crosses into the cell but into the brain), is truly a God-given gift to those crying out for answers. Removing neurotoxins that have bioaccumulated in the brain over the years is the key to why so many people have unexplainable symptoms, illnesses, and "have tried everything" and still don't feel well. It is also an answer for the hormone havoc epidemic that exists today, even in our children. Remove the interference, and the body will do the healing: This is where sincere hope lies, not in man's manufactured chemicals.

Preventing retox, or autointoxication as explain above, throughout the entire process is necessary. Most toxins move from the cell to the liver and dump into the gut. Once in the gut, toxins must transport out of the body so that they do not reabsorb. Autointoxication causes dangerous symptoms and stays a common occurrence in most downstream detox programs, another reason that using true binders during detox is critical to get results safely. Again, health will only return once cellular functions improve via the 5Rs, and real detox agents that can pull toxins from the cell, are used to avoid toxin redistribution.

This situation goes beyond being fat adapted or having a good fast. Cellular detox saves lives, as it did mine and thousands of others. We have hundreds of testimonies, including my own and many of the doctors trained in this process. You can go to my website, *www.drpompa.com*, for more information on my detox protocols.

Chapter 9

ADDITIONAL STEMNOMIC SOLUTIONS: TAKING STEM CELL FUNCTION TO THE NEXT LEVEL

Recall that the concept of Stemnomics is the use of therapeutic strategies that enhance the production and use of stem cells. Herbal medicine can do just that; help raise our stem cell production and viability.

Herbal medicine is the original form of medicine, and is still widely used across the globe to this day. Herbology (including botanicals, animal products, and minerals) was the original form of supplement, and the root of many modern pharmaceutical drugs actually can be traced back to plants as well. We find uses of herbal medicines in almost all societies and cultures, in fact their use to treat diseases dates back over 5,000 years. Today, nearly one-third of Americans use herbs to treat a wide range of conditions including allergies, asthma, eczema, premenstrual syndrome, rheumatoid arthritis, fibromyalgia, migraines, menopausal symptoms, chronic fatigue, irritable bowel syndrome, and cancer.

For over 3,000 years, the people of Asia have been using a wide variety of natural matter and have developed a sophisticated system to harness plant wisdom both for healing and preventative healthcare. Asian herbalism is founded on the principle that true healthcare is rooted in preventative practices, and that it should not be pursued as simply an after-thought once someone is sick. In Chinese and Ayurvedic medicine, these regenerative and healing herbs are called tonic or supplemental herbs.[1] In the West, we call these same herbs adaptogens, due to their ability to help the human body to adapt to stressors both inside the body and externally as we navigate life.

HOW TONIC HERBS ENHANCE STEM CELL ACTIVITY

Although indigenous people around the world have traditionally consumed tonic herbs as foods, they are really in a whole separate class of plant and animal materials than the standard nutrient-dense foods that most of us will find in the produce section of our local health food store. While standard foods are the foundation of our sustenance because they have basic macronutrients (proteins, fats, carbohydrates) and micronutrients (vitamins, minerals) that fuel the body and rebuild our tissues, tonic herbs are most of the time vastly more complex in their chemical makeup.

Most herbs used in herbal medicine have a wide variety of active ingredients, chemicals, or constituents that have a deep, multi-layered effect on all the systems in the body. This complexity gives them higher therapeutic action than standard foods and allows them to stimulate regeneration in the body.[2] They can orchestrate the creation and activation of new stem cells through the complex signaling capability of their vast array of active constituents. The regenerative effects of these premier herbs never come from the linear action of one single constituent, but from the combination of all the active parts in the plants living matrix.[3]

When an individual consumes a medicinal herb over time, it's this balanced matrix that synchronizes with the living, regenerative matrix inside the person's own body and creates greater balance, stimulates regenerative processes, and strengthens the body's overall health. So, the innate intelligence of the plant organism works in symbiosis with the innate intelligence of the human organism when a person brings it into their body, and this could be because both organisms are living systems that originate from the same large living system, which is the natural ecology of the planet.

A notable example of this is Panax Ginseng. Ginseng is a perennial plant that has used as a popular herbal medicine for thousands of years in traditional Chinese medicine (TCM). It is well known for its regenerative properties that promote vitality, prolong life, and show effects against a variety of conditions, including depression, diabetes, fatigue, aging, inflammation, and internal degeneration.[4] Ginseng has been shown in many scientific studies to promote the self-renewal, proliferation, and differentiation of stem cells (creation of new stem cells and new tissues).[5] Besides ginseng, there are several other powerful stem cell proliferators from traditional Chinese and Ayurvedic Medicine scientifically validated such as:[6]

- Prepared Rehmannia (Rehmannia glutinosa)[7]
- Prepared He Shou Wu (Polygonum Multiflorum)[8]
- Salvia root (Salvia Miltiorrhiza)[9]
- Wild Astragalus Root (Astragalus propinquus)[10]
- Aged Wild Red Panax Ginseng (matured for eight years minimum)[11]
- Deer Antler Velvet (Cervus Nippon)

The science around how specific ingredients stimulate stem cell enhancement is strong, and I became excited about creating a product that would help the average person, whether sick and trying to regain their health, prevent age-related disease, or stay healthy longer. Used this product during daily intermittent fasting, extended fasting, or daily without fasting.

I teamed up with Cameron George, credited at the beginning of the book, on this project and started sourcing the ingredients only to find that most had contamination or were not active enough to work. However, after months of thoroughly investigating countless suppliers from around the world, he pulled together some of the highest quality ingredients available anywhere, which quickly met all our strict quality standards and far surpassed all our expectations.

Using these ingredients, we created two separate products, each of which supports one of the two bodily phases of the Recycle/Renewal principle.

Cell CLR is a product that enhances cellular autophagy (the Recycle phase) and supports the body's ability to break down unhealthy cells and stored body fat, to convert them into usable energy as fuel. Cell CLR is made up of a combination of nutrients and herbs that many scientific studies show promotes higher levels of this cellular autophagy in the body. We like to use this product during fasting windows or keto adaptation to take autophagy to the next level and rid the body of as many old or damaged cells as possible.

Cell ReNu is a multi-pathway stem cell enhancement product that supports many critical mechanisms of the body's natural regenerative process. (the Renewal phase). Cell ReNu is a combination of nutrients and herbs that have been shown in many scientific studies to promote healthy function and growth of new stem cells in the body. We like to use this product during feeding windows or refeeding after a fast to feed newly formed stem cells to maximize their ability to renew tissues in the body.

RED LIGHT THERAPY

This amazing therapy can increase your stem cells and can be used after stem cell injections to activate the stem cells in areas of injury or damage. The new cells are attracted to the energy this therapy creates.

We've talked about the dangers of blue light exposure.[12] Red light therapy is very amazing in terms of continued healing strategies. There's a significant difference between the effects that light has on the body as you move across the spectrum of wavelengths. Red spectrum light is a notable example of this: It's as beneficial to the body as overexposure to blue light is harmful. Some effects of red light exposure include:

- Higher energy levels and some have reported better sleep after a nightly light therapy session.[13]

- Improved skin tone, including a reduction in the appearance of wrinkles and stretch marks, probably via stimulation of new collagen growth.[14]

- Increased stem cell production. [15]

- Helping to clear up skin breakouts such as include or eczema.[16]
- Improving circulation.[17]
- Stimulates testosterone production.[18]
- Improvement in age-related macular degeneration.[19]
- Boosting lymph movement through the body.
- Promoting wound healing.[20]
- Reduction in loss of muscle and bone tissue (You can imagine why NASA was specifically interested in this benefit).[21]
- Improved cognitive and motor function, particularly successful in dealing with neurological dysfunction or traumatic brain injury.[22]
- Wound care, reduction in recovery times after strenuous workouts.[23]
- Decreasing free radical formation and inflammation inside the cell.[24]
- Helping with pain management.[25]
- May reduce anxiety by having an overall calming effect on the body.[26]

Most of the benefits of red light therapy come from its ability to recharge your mitochondria, which are the batteries of every cell in your body. These light frequencies supply photons to your mitochondria, which is what allows them to make this extra energy in the form of ATP. Everything works better when these batteries charge. Therefore, such a wide variety of benefits derive from exposing yourself to these specific light frequencies.

In a recent *Cellular Healing TV* episode, I interviewed Joovv founders, Scott Nelson, and Justin Strahan. Along with their wives, Justin and Scott created Joovv; a company focused on bringing superior phototherapy products that you can use in the comfort of your own home. As experts on red light therapy, Scott and Justin shared their knowledge on how red light photobiomodulation works and how to choose a high-quality red light for the best therapeutic results.

The Joovv light is the most reliable and effective device I've come across. It delivers clinical-grade power in a practical home unit that can be used daily and will last for years to come. For best results, Justin and Scott recommend positioning your Joovv approximately six inches from the area on your body you intend to treat. The recommended default treatment time is ten minutes per treatment area, which will result in a clinically proven effect dosage. Clinical studies have shown that this combination of distance and power is effective for producing health benefits in both superficial and deep tissues.

PULSED ELECTROMAGNETIC FIELD THERAPY (PEMF)

Pulsed Electromagnetic Field Therapy (PEMF or PEMT) is a treatment for various injuries, bone-related conditions, and pain that does not cause any trauma or added pain. This non-invasive treatment works a pulsing electromagnetic field that varies in intensity and frequency. These pulsed electromagnetic frequencies have been shown to accelerate healing and restore the body's natural healing potential. It has been applied clinically to promote wound healing by reducing inflammation while regenerating tissue through stem cell enhancement.[27] Unlike many modern medical innovations, pulsed electromagnetic field therapy has little to no side-effects, which makes it tolerable even to individuals in fragile states of health. Here's how it works.

When there is a disturbance in the cells electromagnetic energy field, a cascade of problems ensue. The cells metabolism is imparied, which eventually triggers a disease process that eventually prevents the cell from performing its natural self-repairing. When a cell loses its ability to recover, we see the drastic rise of modern chronic illnesses plaguing the modern world.

Pulsed electromagnetic field therapy targets this imbalanced chemistry within the cell. The medical solenoid device generates low-frequency magnetic fields, which safely pass through the body and penetrate every single cell, tissue, organ, and bone. By doing so, these unaltered frequencies are able to stimulate the body's natural electrical and chemical processes, thus improving the cell metabolism and regenerative ability. As the cells regain their health, they can then return to their ability to repair tissue and heal the body.[28]

The magnetic field is generated by an electrical current runs through a copper coil. There are a wide variety of PEMF devices on the market, all of which have a *slightly* different effect. Out of all the devices available, there are three in particular that I recommend, based on the greatest results I have experienced both directly and with my clients.[29]

- Pulse Centers makes the most powerful PEMF device on the market that can stimulate stem cells and direct them to the area of injury. It is the go-to device in most clinical practices, including mine.

- The BEMER (Bio Electro Magnetic Energy Regulation)—This is a full body mat developed in Switzerland. It is different from standard PEMF devices. It uses a unique patented signal to enhance what's called microcirculation, which is made up of all the smallest blood vessels that deliver oxygen and nutrients to the deepest tissues of the body and carry waste away from them for elimination. It works to enhance all the other therapies and nutritional strategies that a person is already using, including the delivery of stem cells to damaged areas. You can find a local practitioner who offers this therapy or buy one yourself for home use at a more significant expense.

- ICES systems—Robert Dennis, a scientist who included some original PEMF systems that NASA used in the late 90s created these systems. These are PEMF devices that were included through years of comprehensive research and are of the highest quality for standard PEMF devices. They are portable units, which are much more affordable than most others, and are more effective.

All three devices help to support the function and delivery of stem cells in tissues all over the body. They are all effective, especially when used within the multi-therapeutic approach.

HYPERBARIC OXYGEN THERAPY (HBOT)

Hyperbaric oxygen therapy (HBOT) is a medical treatment that promotes the body's natural ability to heal through the inhalation of pure oxygen inside a pressurized chamber. It is primarily used[30] as an overall supportive therapy for recovery from a vast array of different injuries and illnesses such as:

- Traumatic Brain Injury

- PTSD

- Depression and Anxiety

- Chronic Fatigue Syndrome

- Autism

- Stroke

- Multiple sclerosis

- Burn injuries

- Systemic and skin infections

- Sudden vision loss

Under normal circumstances, oxygen transports throughout the body only by red blood cells. With HBOT, the added pressure dissolves oxygen into all the body's fluids—the plasma, spinal fluid, the lymph, and the bone—and carries it to areas where there is impaired circulation. By doing so, the extra oxygen can reach the damaged tissues, and the body can support its healing process. However, the increased oxygen availability is not the only reason for the amazing effects of this therapy.

In recent years, research proves that the increased pressure in hyperbaric oxygen has a profound effect on the body's genetic expression.[31] A 2008 study found that a single hyperbaric treatment turns on or turns off over 8,000 genes in the twenty-four hours following the therapy. Furthermore, they found that the genes that turned on are anti-inflammatory genes[32] and genes coded for growth and repair hormones. The genes turned off were the pro-inflammatory genes and coded for cell death.[33] Multiple studies have also shown that HBOT seems to activate stem cells and mobilize them to damaged tissues. Together with the massive growth hormone rise, this is one of the most powerful therapies available for anti-aging and re-generation.

HBOT is widely available today in the U.S. and other countries around the world. Almost every major hospital has a hyperbaric unit with medical grade chambers. However, getting this therapy in a hospital is expensive and frankly unnecessary in most cases. Finding a stand-alone clinic in your area will run you about one-tenth of the cost, usually about $150-$250 per one-hour treatment. Some people with more acute conditions may require only a few treatments.

As for chronic conditions and general anti-aging, individuals may receive help from dozens or sometimes hundreds of treatments be-cause the effects are cumulative. In these cases, the most cost-effective approach is to rent or invest in a portable home unit. The portable chamber I most recommend is from a company called Oxy Health. These chambers are thoroughly tested for safety and efficacy and made without the use of any chemical adhesives, particularly important because any contaminants that out-gas within the cham-ber can become hyper absorbed in your tissues along with the oxy-gen. Getting or renting a portable chamber can save much money over time and is the most practical way for the average person to receive the effects of this amazing therapy.

STEM CELL THERAPY

Finally, here are the big guns. Stem cell therapies are a class of medi-cal procedures that involve injecting live stem cells into various places in the body to stimulate the regenerative process directly. They are being used both domestically and abroad to help in the treatment of a massive variety of different conditions such as:

- Sports-related and overuse injuries such as torn muscles, liga-ments [34]

- Chronic pain and arthritis[35]

- Traumatic brain injury[36]

- Congestive heart failure[37]

- Spinal cord injury[38]

- Parkinson's disease[39]

- Alzheimer's disease and dementia[40]

- Autoimmune conditions[41]

- Diabetes[42]

- Kidney disease[43]

- Macular degeneration[44]

- Also applied for general anti-aging[45]

Theoretically, stem cell therapies could help with every single condition, since cells are inevitably involved in every single disease model in the human body. Medical experts across a vast array of different specialties have long predicted them to be the future "holy grail" of medicine. I think this is true and I believe that in addition to stem cell injections, the future of chronic disease care will have to include strategies, like those that I've laid out in this book's seven-week plan. These strategies optimize the body's internal terrain and better prepare it to receive regenerative therapies.

When I spoke of the Recycle/Renewal Principle in the Introduction, I explained the critical role that recycling (autophagy) plays in cellular renewal (creation of new stem cells), comparing it to the necessity of having to break down an old damaged house to build a new one in its place. Just like autophagy is necessary to maximize your body's endogenous production of stem cells, so it's also necessary to maximize the clinical results that a patient can receive from exogenous stem cell injections.

Therefore, I believe that the real future of medicine for chronic disease will be a combination of functional medicine (terrain preparation) and regenerative medicine (stem cell-related therapies). It's when we apply both fields together that we can see the most miraculous clinical results even today.

However, why would a person following this book's plan want or need to seek out stem cell therapy? Doesn't the plan itself already stimulate stem cell production? Yes, and the strategies outlined in this book should always be the foundational approach to healing and regeneration. However, in many circumstances, there can be limitations to how much healing can occur from lifestyle and supplemental strategies alone. In these circumstances, stem cell therapy is the single most powerful adjunct to my program that exists today. It is most effective when applied after all the strategies in my program are in place for some time; especially proper detoxification and fasting. It works synergistically when combined with any of the therapies or modalities mentioned previously.

My story makes this point well. Years ago, I damaged my lower back, severely herniated a disc, and tore many of the stabilizing ligaments. It healed without surgery, but in the years following, I would manage to re-injure it, or it would just go out for no clear reason. As I aged, this happened increasingly. My viable stems cells were dropping regardless of my healthy lifestyle and fasting.

The fasting, diet variation and cellular detoxification turned back my cellular age as determined by a telomere *test*. These test measures telomeres, which are the only biological clock we know. My first cellular age test was 64 because of my illness and mercury toxicity. My actual age as of this writing is 53, and recent testing shows my cellular age to be 43.

The point is there was little blood flow in my disc, and combined with the natural lowering of viable stem cell as we age, I needed help. The stem cell injections change my life. To watch my procedure, you can watch the interview with Dr. Harry Adelson, ND (*Cellular Healing TV episode #220*) and Dr. Ahvie Herskowitz, MD, (*Cellular Healing TV episodes #227 and #240*) who also did some amazing stem cell work with me.

For information regarding stem cells and many other conditions such as immune system, neurodegenerative, autoimmune and autism, watch *Cellular Healing TV episode 263*, where I interviewed Dr. Raphael Gonzales from Rehealth Clinic, in Cancun, Mexico. They are doing some amazing things with new stem cell technologies and Natural Killer cells.

There are four main groups of people who might be interested in receiving the added benefit of stem cell therapy.

- The elderly.
- Those with compromised health.
- Those with chronic injuries that are not healing because of low viable stem cells because of toxicity or age, which was my case.
- Those wanting anti-aging effects and total health optimization.

TYPES OF STEM CELL TREATMENTS

The next step is to investigate the types of therapies that are available and to find a practicing physician who specializes in them. As I addressed earlier in the book; not all stem cells are created equal. There are diverse types of stem cells, and therefore, many types of stem cell therapies that have cells from a variety of sources. All these therapies fall into two major categories: Autologous and Allogeneic treatments.

AUTOLOGOUS

Autologous procedures involve using stem cells harvested from the patient's body, which includes the safest choice so that there no risk of any adverse reactions or other side effects. Although we can extract stem cells from virtually all tissues, most physicians doing autologous treatments are harvesting the cells from either the patient's bone marrow, fat, or peripheral blood.

Most of the cells harvested from these areas are "adult stem cells" known as MSCs (Mesenchymal Stem Cells) which means they are stem cells that arose in the body after the embryonic stage of human development and are therefore less potent in their regenerative abilities than much younger embryonic stem cells.

MSCs work differently when injected into the body. Unlike embryonic stem cells, that can become any cell type in the body directly replacing damaged cells, MSCs primarily work by seeking out areas of damage and secreting signals that stimulate cells to repair themselves. We call this process, paracrine signaling.

Although they are not as potent as younger stem cells, they have still been shown to be very effective clinically. Bone marrow and fat are the richest sources of stem cells in the body, and treatments that have cells from these areas are comprised mainly of MSCs.[46] You can find more information on bone marrow and fat stem cell treatments provided by Dr. Harry Adelson at www.docereclinics.com.

Bone Marrow: For bone marrow treatments, it is important to understand that harvesting for stem cell therapy is vastly simpler than bone marrow harvesting for transfusion for cancer therapies. It requires a relatively small amount of bone marrow from a single puncture site. They extract the bone marrow using a local anesthetic, then further process removing the stem cells and injecting them back into the patient. The procedure is considered extremely safe, and is much less painful than you might imagine. It usually takes under ten minutes and causes only a mild soreness afterward that lasts only a few days.

Fat: Treatments using cells harvested from fat (adipose tissue) are a remarkably uncomplicated process called lipoaspiration. It is important to understand that lipoaspiration differs vastly from liposuction. A plastic surgeon performs liposuction, removing up to 6,000 ml (6 liters) of fat, for a cosmetic result. Lipoaspiration, on the other hand, requires a small amount of local anesthetic and a hypodermic-sized needle is used to remove a fraction of the amount (about 1/100th, or 60 ml). The entire process takes around fifteen minutes.

Peripheral Blood: Some physicians are harvesting stem cells from their patient's own blood for autologous treatments. In recent years they have discovered that human blood has stem cells that are even more potent than MSCs called VSELS (Very Small Embryonic-like Stem Cells). Just as the name implies, they are embryonic-like, which means they also can directly become and replace any cell type in the body and is exciting for a couple of reasons. First, harvesting stem cells from the blood is by far the easiest and least invasive way to obtain them from the patient's body. It just requires a simple blood draw. Second, VSELS could might be far more potent than MSCs and offer extra support in conditions that involve severely damaged tissues such as brain and spinal cord injuries. VSELS may play a significant role in the future of stem cell medicine.

ALLOGENIC

These are procedures that involve using stem cells that come from a donor. The main reason to choose this option would be to obtain younger, healthier cells from another person when the patient's cells are compromised. Very elderly or sick individuals would be good candidates for this procedure. Physicians using allogeneic treatments also use stem cells that come from a variety of different tissue sources.

Umbilical Cord: This is the most commonly used source of stem cells in allogeneic treatments today. These treatments are mainly MSCs but are young and therefore more potent than most cells found in an adult patient's tissues. Clinics around the world are buying umbilical cord stem cell products harvested from healthy C-sectioned births and donated by the mothers. They are processed, purified, and screened thoroughly for every possible known infectious disease and administered to patients in the form of simple injections. Although these cells are coming from a donor, they don't appear to cause any acute immune reactions because they come from tissue that is "universal" not technically mom or baby. Cells are neutral; otherwise, either mom or baby would reject them during pregnancy. Treatments using these cells generally appear to be safe. However, not yet thoroughly studied, we can't say for sure that there are no potential side effects long term.

Embryonic: Most of us know the controversy centered on embryonic stem cells started in the early 2000s and continuing today because many people believe that aborted fetal tissue is the source of these harvested cells. This belief is false. Today most embryonic cells come from in-vitro fertilization. These cells are extremely potent and, as I mentioned before, can directly become any cell type in the body. Because they are foreign cells that are not universal, they might turn into cancer cells or cause immune reactions when used clinically. For these reasons, they are illegal to use in the United States but are available in many countries around the world. Many physicians are starting to look to VSELS as a potential future alternative to these cells.

Exosomes: If stem cells are the future of medicine, and I believe they are, exosomes could be the future of stem cells. Although they are not a cell at all, they are communication molecules that cells use to carry messages from cell to cell and even activate healing. When first discovered they were thought to be cellular rubbish, but now scientists have discovered that they are the active healing component to stem cells, meaning this gives rise to the healing that stem cells do. Not too many years ago, scientists thought the healing from stem cells was the cells turning into the tissue where they were injected or migrated to, and then becoming healthier tissue in that area. We call this process differentiation.

Today they realize this is a small part of what takes place. Most of the healing is done by what is called a paracrine effect, which means the stem cells release exosomes, and they communicate with your resident stem cells in that area and signal them to start the healing.

So, what if we can isolate these exosomes and do not need the actual stem cells? Stem cells might have other problems because they carry the DNA of the donor. The exosomes are potentially more powerful as well because they carry the vitality of a young cell ready to drive a significant healing response. Welcome to the new world of exosomes. I had these amazing healing VSELS injected into me a few times with impressive results, and I can tell you it's easier than harvesting your own from fat or bone marrow and safer than getting bad cells. I believe it's the future of stem cells and whether or not we are there yet, this is a great option if you are looking to up your healing game.

FROM THE SCIENTIST HIMSELF

I asked scientist and stem cell researcher Dr. Rafael Gonzalez to describe the science around this emerging topic to give you a more scientific view of what they are, how they work, and the future potential. Extracellular vesicles (EVs) were first discovered over 50 years ago in plasma. All cells and biological fluids contain these mini "packets" of information essential for the body to function daily. There are three main types of EVs based on their mechanism of release and size. Here we will briefly overview the smallest of these messenger packets, exosomes which have been of much interest and hype as of late.

Exosomes are small and produced within cells. All cells produce exosomes as they are essential for cell-cell communication, survival, and maintaining cellular health and extracellular integrity. They are approximately $1/1000^{th}$ of the size of a cell. Exosomes are cargos of information that can come in the form of micro RNAs (miRNAs), proteins, or lipids (fats). Interestingly, they have a similar lipid membrane composition like cells, which serves as a protection mechanism when released from inside the cell. Following the release to the extracellular matrix, the cargo gets delivered, or travels to fuse with neighboring cells and then delivers that important cargo. To keep a healthy physiological environment, exosomes are produced within cells and released for use by neighboring cells or production of any needed proteins within the environment—collagen, growth factors, and chemical messengers. Moreover, exosomes are secreted in higher abundance when cells are stressed; which is our body's natural healing response to a problem that needs addressing.

The regenerative medicine sector has an immense interest in using exosomes for healing and repair, of isolating them from stem cells and other tissues that have been shown to have regenerative medicine properties. Moreover, we understand that adult stem cells act in a paracrine manner (secrete exosomes and proteins) that affect neighboring cells to heal and repair. Therefore, the interest in this field is to isolate these cargo packets or effectors and deliver them to sites of benefit so they can start the healing. It is still to be confirmed with large scale clinical studies if exosomes will be as successful as stem cells. Stay tuned for the verdict.

CONCLUSION

Today there are millions of people suffering from the symptoms of premature aging and chronic degenerative diseases. With that, there is a huge need for tools and strategies that individuals can use to maximize their body's ability to maintain optimal health and vitality. This situation has given rise to the field of applied Stemnomics (the use of therapeutic strategies that enhance the production and utilization of stem cells). The reason I authored this book was to pull together all the forefront strategies that my colleagues and I find the most effective and credible and which maximize the body's stem cell activity.

As I stated in this book's introduction, my core philosophy is to remove the interference, and the body will do the healing. However, with or without interference, the body still needs viable stem cells to orchestrate the healing process and renew itself. The problem today that many are facing is that toxins, traumas, age, and stress deplete us of viable stem cells. Our ability to recover and heal diminishes with each of these strikes we have against us. It's not normal to have the aches and pains, loss of energy, and brain fog that so many have today, and this is because of the loss of these stem cells and brings about premature aging.

Over the years, I have found that there is nothing more powerful than relying on the body's innate intelligence to do the healing. We know so little of how the body works. There is a phrase, "the more we know, the more we realize how little we know." The body knows what to do if we remove the interference and allow the power within to unleash. All true healing comes from inside out, not outside in, and this is how I got my life back and how thousands of others who find their way to one of my trained practitioners do.

Over the years, a growing group of practitioners from around the world are combining the True Cellular Detox and the fasting principles in *Beyond Fasting*, relying entirely on the innate healing wisdom of the body. The results have been extraordinary. I hope the information in this book will empower you and provide you with the practical means take control of your health, prevent disease, and reach your full human potential to be the best version of yourself. If you are a practitioner and want to join up with our group and take these principles to a hurting world and share your results, please visit *www.stemnomicrevolution.com*.

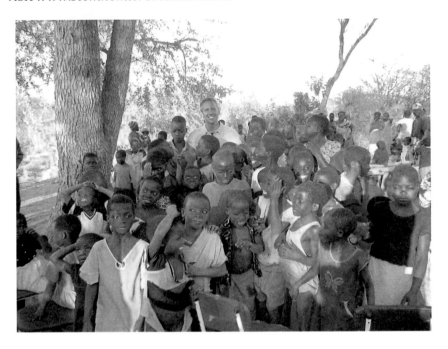

Dr. Daniel Pompa while visiting Africa.

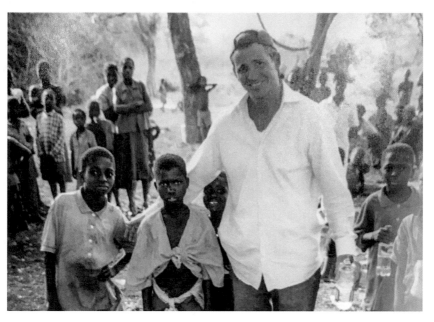

Dr. Daniel Pompa while visiting Africa.

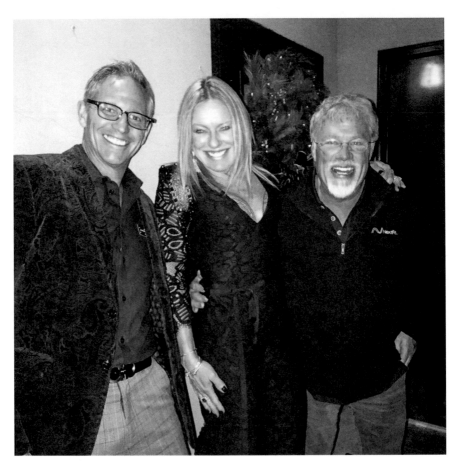

Dr. Daniel and Merily Pompa, and Jeff Hayes

MEAL PLANS AND RECIPES

QUALITY FIRST!

I cannot overstate the importance of sourcing high-quality organic food. For the body to thrive, it needs nourishment with real, whole, unprocessed foods that will not add to the toxic burden of the body. Produce and animal products that have led an unnatural life (be it sprayed with pesticides, or

injected with hormones or antibiotics) will pass down these poisons to you, and force your body to either process them out, burdening your liver and organs, or more likely store them in the body's tissues, organs, and fat stores.

For the body to produce new stem cells efficiently and effectively, seek food in its natural, organic state. For meat, seek organic, pasture-raised meat; animals that have led natural lives in pastures under the sunshine is not only ethical, but it will provide your body with nutrient-dense food to thrive.

REMINDERS: Choose raw nuts and cheese, grass-fed meat, pastured, free- range and cage-free eggs, and no-hormones sources whenever possible. Avoid farm-raised and Atlantic fish. Avoid hydrogenated, partially hydrogenated, and vegetable oils, including canola oil. Use cold- pressed oils. Use ORGANIC when possible.

For convenience, we have omitted repeating the following words in the ingredient lists of the recipes, but they are inferred:

Organic

Grass-fed

Pasture-raised

Free-range

Farm-fresh

Cage-free

No hormones added

Raw

HIGHER CARBOHYDRATE OPTIONS MEALS
FOR WEEK ONE AND ANY FEAST DAYS

NOTE: Italicized items can be found in the *Meal Plans and Recipes* section.

Breakfast

- Poached eggs with sweet potato hash, mushrooms, and avocado
- Breakfast frittata with bacon, sweet potato, spinach, and feta
- Sweet potato muffins with lots of butter and cinnamon
- Smoothies—*Super Green Smoothie, Caramel Smoothie, Sweet Potato Almond Butter Smoothie, Ruby Red Zinger Smoothie, Carrot Cake Shake, Nutty Green Smoothie*
- *Banana Pancakes with Homemade Coconut Yogurt and Cinnamon*
- Fried eggs with bacon, home fries, and grilled tomatoes
- Sweet potato protein pancakes with cottage cheese and walnuts
- *Sweet Breakfast Muffins* with banana, sweet potato, nuts, seeds, coconut oil
- Yogurt or kefir with berries and granola or nuts

Lunch

- Salad with fish or chicken and potato mashed with ghee or butter, chives, and parsley
- Crudité platter with raw cheese, figs, and *Beef Liver Pâté*
- *Sweet Potato "Toast"* with avocado, smoked salmon, and sea salt
- Mushroom soup topped with seeds and avocado
- *Carrot Soup Drizzled with Olive Oil and Prosciutto*
- Oven roasted chicken thighs with honey-roasted carrots drizzled with olive oil, sea salt
- Nori rolls with sardines, baked sweet potato, cucumber, sprouts, and peppers
- *Lentils and Warm Vegetable Stir-Fry with Olives, Basil, and Drizzled in Olive Oil*

Dinner

- *Roasted Vegetables Drizzled with Olive Oil, Sea Salt,* medley vegetables - carrots, sweet potato, parsnips, peppers, and broccoli
- Beef with asparagus and *Hasselback Potatoes* with butter
- *Roasted Leg of Lamb with Mint Yogurt* and *Garlic Green Beans* and
- *Sweet Potato Mash*
- *Roast Chicken* with broccoli and *Crispy Sweet Potato Fries*
- Curry chicken on a bed of jasmine rice
- Crispy salmon pan fried in ghee, with charred asparagus and oven roasted beetroot "chips"
- Baked potato loaded with pulled chicken, bacon, cheese, chives, and sour cream
- *Slow-Cooked Braised Beef Cheek Stew* made with potatoes
- *Nacho Salad* with rice

LOWER CARBOHYDRATE OPTIONS FOR ANY MEALS

*Note that feast days should have more carbohydrates.

NOTE: Italicized items can be found in the *Meal Plans and Recipes* section.

Breakfast

- Fried eggs, with grilled halloumi cheese, mushrooms, and avocado
- Frittata, with mushrooms, tomatoes, red and green peppers, feta, and fresh green herbs
- *Omelet*, with grilled asparagus, prosciutto, and cheese
- Smoothies—*Strawberry Mint Smoothie, Green Berry Beauty Smoothie, Probiotic Protein Smoothie Powerhouse Smoothie, Creamy Chocolate Avocado Smoothie, Wild Blueberry Smoothie*
- *Chia Pudding*
- *Chocolate Avocado Pudding*
- Super green and lean omelet with spinach, parsley, leeks, arugula, and avocado
- Optional: Bacon or shredded chicken
- Loaded Mexican-style omelet with shredded chicken, cheese, chives, parsley, coriander, salsa, and sour cream
- Poached eggs on a bed of arugula, with grilled asparagus, avocado, and mushrooms
- Yogurt or kefir with fresh berries, nuts/seeds, with nut butter
- Shakshuka—baked eggs in tomato sauce with mushrooms and herbs

Lunch/Dinner

- Salmon ceviche with avocado and spring onion
- *Oven-Baked Crispy, Spicy Chicken Wings* with raw carrots, celery, and a blue cheese dip

- Beef Tataki with an Asian style slaw
- Sashimi with seaweed salad
- *Avocado Gazpacho*
- *Guacamole* made with sardines, with carrot sticks and another raw vegetable
- Bacon wrapped jalapeños stuffed with cream cheese
- *Spicy Turmeric Roasted Cauliflower*
- *Nacho Salad*
- *Green Soup* topped with bacon bits
- *Green Soup* with avocado, toasted seeds, and drizzled with olive oil
- Barbequed chicken with grilled eggplant and zucchini with *Lemon Tahini Sauce*
- Oven roasted carrots with *Lemon Tahini Sauce*
- *Coconut Wraps* with chicken, shredded carrots, avocado, and cilantro
- *Coconut Wraps* with sardines, avocado, cucumber, and parsley
- Green salad with mackerel, avocado, cucumber, olive oil, lemon juice, and sea salt
- Cucumber, tomato, feta, and olive salad with olive oil
- Roasted asparagus soup drizzled with olive oil and crumbled feta
- *Shaved Zucchini and Fennel Salad* with *Roast Chicken*
- Raw vegetables dipped with red pepper dip and Baba Ganoush
- Big green salad, with beef, tomatoes avocado, olive oil, and lemon juice
- *Beef Mushroom Lettuce Tacos*
- Steak with grilled asparagus, avocado, and charred jalapeños
- *Roast Chicken* with broccoli drizzled in olive oil
- *Cauliflower Crust Pizza* topped with pesto, chicken, and arugula

- Grilled fish with cucumber, feta, tomato, and olive salad
- *Chicken Zoodle Soup*
- *Zucchini Noodles with Pesto and Beef Meatballs*
- Eggplant Parmesan
- *Slow-Cooked Braised Beef Cheek Stew*
- Curry chicken on a bed of greens
- *Roasted Leg of Lamb with Mint Yogurt* and *Garlic Green Beans*
- Oven-baked salmon with roasted fennel and carrots
- *Cauliflower Mash*
- Zucchini noodles with shredded chicken, grilled peppers, and mushrooms
- Chicken Pad Thai with shirataki noodles

KETOSIS-FRIENDLY RECIPES
LOW CARBOHYDRATE
BREAKFAST

Crispy Oven-Baked Bacon

High-quality bacon is nutrient dense and a great source of healthy fats. Look for bacon that is organic, pasture-raised and has NO added sugar, sulfites, or preservatives. Opt for uncured, reduced-sodium center cut bacon. READ THE LABEL!

INGREDIENTS

- 1 package of non-GMO bacon strips

INSTRUCTIONS

1. Preheat oven to 400° F.
2. Place the bacon strips lined up, side-by-side on a baking tray.
3. Cook on the second highest oven rack for 10 minutes and flip strips to the other side.
4. Cook for another 5–10 minutes, watching to see when they have reached the desired level of crispness.
5. Remove from oven and place on a paper towel to remove the excess fat, which will ensure they crisp up before consumption.

TIP

- DO NOT DISCARD THE BACON FAT! With high-quality bacon, the extra fat in the tray is perfect for cooking. Put the lard into a glass jar and store it in the fridge for future cooking, particularly great for roasting vegetables.

Homemade Coconut Yogurt

INGREDIENTS

- 2 13.5-ounce cans of full-fat coconut cream
- 4 capsules of probiotic—not a prebiotic/probiotic combo
- 2 teaspoons gelatin—optional, for a thicker consistency
- 3 tablespoons collagen—optional, for more protein content
- 1 large mason jar, wooden spoon, clean cloth, rubber band

INSTRUCTIONS

1. Sterilize your mason jar and utensils with boiling water and set aside to dry.

2. Put the coconut cream into a saucepan, stir while you bring it to a simmer only, then remove from heat.

3. If using gelatin and collagen, stir in while hot.

4. Let the coconut cream cool until it is room temperature.

5. Fill one-half of the mason jar with the coconut cream, break the four probiotic capsules into the mix and stir well with the wooden spoon.

6. Add the rest of the coconut cream to the mason jar and then stir again with the wooden spoon.

7. Use the rubber band to secure the cloth over the top of the jar and leave it in the oven for 48 hours, with the oven light turned on.

8. Refrigerate for at least 6 hours before consuming. It will firm up in the fridge.

TIPS

- Make sure you use a wooden or plastic spoon to stir probiotic (not metal).
- If you use a probiotic capsule that also has a prebiotic, it will not ferment.

- Use full-fat coconut cream, not coconut milk, which creates a liquid yogurt.

- If the coconut cream is too hot when you mix the probiotic, the live cultures of the probiotic will die.

- Fermentation requires a stable temperature plus a slightly warm environment. Store your filled mason jar in the oven, with the temperature off, but the oven light on. The oven light produces enough heat within the oven to ferment the yogurt, but not kill off the probiotic.

- The Homemade Coconut Yogurt may separate, which is normal. You can stir it up, or to keep it thicker, put it in the refrigerator separated, then consume the creamy top layer.

- You may remove the yogurt from your oven incubator after only 24 hours, but longer will produce a more fermented taste while giving the probiotic enough time to proliferate.

Chocolate Avocado Pudding or Fudge Popsicles

INGREDIENTS

- 2 ripe avocados
- 2 heaping tablespoons cacao powder or cocoa or carob
- ½ 13.5-ounce can of full-fat coconut cream
- 3 heaping tablespoons collagen powder
- ½ teaspoon of cinnamon
- A pinch of sea salt

Optional: One teaspoon of your preferred superfoods, such as maca, pine pollen, reishi, and chaga.

INSTRUCTIONS

1. Blend all the ingredients in a food processor until smooth. You may need to scrape down the sides and blend again. You can add extra coconut cream until you reach your desired consistency.

Optional: Freeze for 30 minutes for an ice cream-like consistency. Use popsicle molds to create a cold, creamy chocolate fudge treat.

Chia Pudding

INGREDIENTS

- 3 tablespoons of chia seeds
- 1 cup of milk—coconut, almond, cashew, cow

Optional: One-half teaspoon of vanilla, and any superfood of your choice, such as maca, cinnamon, cacao, açai

Toppings of your choice: Coconut, nuts, seeds, cacao nibs, or fruit

Optional: One-half cup of yogurt

INSTRUCTIONS

1. Soak the chia seeds in your choice of milk, preferably overnight to maximize digestion, but a minimum of 10 minutes. Stir once or twice to ensure they all absorb the liquid.

2. Stir in your choice of superfoods to add more nutrition to your Chia Pudding, as well as the yogurt, and top with your preferred toppings.

NOTE: I like to make big batches of Chia Pudding to keep in the fridge and use throughout the week. Keep the ratio of about 3 tablespoons of chia seeds per cup of milk.

IDEAS FOR CHIA PUDDING COMBINATION

- Chocolate Lovers: Soak chia seeds in coconut milk, stir in 1 tablespoon cacao powder, 1 teaspoon maca, a ½ cup of Homemade Coconut Yogurt, and top with shredded coconut and cacao nibs.

- Berry Bliss: Soak chia seeds in cashew milk, stir in 2 tablespoons shredded coconut, 1 teaspoon açai powder, a ½ cup of Homemade Coconut Yogurt, and top with wild blueberries, raspberries, and bee pollen.

- PB&J: Soak chia seeds in almond milk, stir in 2 tablespoons of peanut butter (or almond butter) and 2 tablespoons of sugar-free jam, top with a handful of berries and crushed peanuts.

- Matcha: Soak chia seeds in coconut milk, stir in 1½ teaspoons of matcha powder.

Omelet

Eggs are a nutritious and filling way to start the day, and omelets are a great way to fill your morning with plenty of vegetables, too. The recipe calls for optional milk, which makes the omelet fluffier and larger, but is unnecessary.

INGREDIENTS

- 4 eggs
- 1 tablespoon olive oil, ghee, or butter
- Your choice of vegetables, meat, herbs, and spices
- Sea salt and black pepper, to taste

Optional: ¼ cup of milk or almond milk

INSTRUCTIONS

1. Whisk together the eggs, milk, salt, and pepper.
2. Heat a pan on medium and add the oil or butter to coat the pan.
3. Pour the whisked mixture onto the pan and place your choice of toppings evenly in the egg mixture.
4. Once the egg starts to cook, and the edges of the omelet crisp up, use a spatula to fold the omelet in half.
5. Cook for another minute or so on each side, until it becomes golden brown.

IDEAS FOR OMELET COMBINATIONS

- Red pepper, mushroom, ham, and gruyere
- Tomato, green pepper, olives, and feta
- Salami, chili, avocado, and parsley

Creamy Chocolate Avocado Smoothie

INGREDIENTS

- ½ avocado, frozen
- 1–2 cups of cauliflower—steamed and then frozen
- 1½ cups nut milk—almond or coconut
- 2 tablespoons cacao powder
- 1 tablespoon coconut butter
- 1 teaspoon cinnamon

Optional: One scoop of collagen powder or protein powder

INSTRUCTIONS

1. Place all the ingredients in a blender and blend on high until smooth.

Wild Blueberry Smoothie

INGREDIENTS

- 2 cups of cauliflower—steamed and then frozen
- ¼ of an avocado, frozen
- 1 cup wild blueberries, frozen
- 1½ cups nut milk—almond or coconut
- 1 heaping tablespoon nut butter of your choice
- 1 teaspoon cinnamon

Optional: One scoop of collagen powder or protein powder

INSTRUCTIONS

1. Place all the ingredients in a blender and blend on high until smooth.

Strawberry Mint Smoothie

INGREDIENTS

- 1 13.5-ounce can of full-fat coconut milk, unsweetened
- 1 12-ounce bag frozen, strawberries (or fresh)
- 1 small bunch of mint
- 1-2 cups chilled, ginger tea (or filtered water to thin)
- 1 tablespoon collagen powder
- ½ teaspoon cinnamon
- ½ teaspoon turmeric
- 1 teaspoon of sea salt

INSTRUCTIONS

1. Add all ingredients, except collagen, to the blender and mix until smooth.
2. Add collagen and incorporate at low speed.

Purple Power Smoothie

INGREDIENTS

- 1 13.5-ounce can of full-fat coconut milk, unsweetened
- 1 chopped beet
- 1 cup frozen blueberries
- 1 teaspoon maca powder
- 1 teaspoon cinnamon
- 1 tablespoon collagen powder
- ½ teaspoon of sea salt

INSTRUCTIONS

1. Add all ingredients, except collagen, to the blender and mix until smooth.
2. Add collagen and incorporate at low speed.

Green Berry Beauty Smoothie

INGREDIENTS

- 1 13.5-ounce can of full-fat coconut milk
- 1 bag frozen strawberries
- 1 cup kale, lightly steamed
- 1 teaspoon pure vanilla extract
- 1 tablespoon raw honey (optional)
- 1 tablespoon collagen powder
- Pinch of sea salt

INSTRUCTIONS

1. Put all ingredients in a high-speed blender and mix until smooth.

Probiotic Protein Powerhouse Smoothie

INGREDIENTS

- 1 13.5-ounce can of full-fat coconut milk
- 1 bag frozen raspberries
- 1 whole, pastured raw eggs
- 2 capsules high-potency probiotic
- 1-2 scoops glutamine powder

INSTRUCTIONS

1. Empty contents of capsules and put all ingredients in a high-speed blender.
2. Blend on LOW until smooth.

KETOSIS-FRIENDLY RECIPES LOW CARBOHYDRATE
LUNCH AND DINNER

Oven-Baked, Crispy, Spicy Chicken Wings

INGREDIENTS

- 1–2 pounds of chicken wings/drumsticks
- 2 tablespoons olive, avocado, or coconut oil
- 3 tablespoons of turmeric powder
- 1 tablespoon of paprika
- A pinch of cayenne pepper
- Sea salt and black pepper, to taste

INSTRUCTIONS

1. Preheat oven to 400° F.

2. Place chicken wings and oil in a bowl and toss to coat the chicken.

3. Add turmeric, paprika, and cayenne and toss again until it covers the wings (use more spice if necessary).

4. Place the wings on a baking tray, lined with parchment paper, so they are not touching each other, and place tray on the second highest rack in the oven.

5. Bake for 10 minutes, flip the wings to the other side, bake another 10 minutes, and flip again. Repeat one more time for each side. Total cooking time is around 40 minutes, but since wings vary in size, keep an eye on them.

6. Season with fresh black pepper and sea salt.

Beef Mushroom Lettuce Tacos

INGREDIENTS

- 2 pounds of grass-fed beef
- 1 tablespoon dried rosemary
- 1 teaspoon dried sage
- 1 teaspoon of sea salt
- 1 teaspoon black pepper
- 1 tablespoon olive, coconut, or avocado oil
- Two handfuls of mushrooms, diced
- 1 head of romaine lettuce
- 1 ripe avocado
- ¼ red onion
- Sauerkraut

INSTRUCTIONS

- Sauté the diced mushrooms in oil, add the rosemary, sage, salt, and pepper.
- Sauté until all the mushrooms are golden brown.
- With mushrooms still in the pan, add all the ground beef, and using a wooden spoon, chop the beef to spread evenly over the pan. Continue to mix the beef and mushrooms until the beef is cooked through (all brown).
- Assemble your tacos with the beef/mushroom mix, avocado, sauerkraut, and red onion.

TIP

- DO NOT DISCARD THE BEEF FAT! If you read the bacon recipe, you'll know that the leftover fat from cooking high-quality fatty meat is full of nutrients. Strain the fat to remove any left of beef or herbs and store it in a glass jar in your fridge for future use.

Zucchini Noodles with Pesto and Beef Meatballs

INGREDIENTS

- ½ pound of grass-fed, pasture-raised ground beef
- 1 zucchini per person
- Two handfuls of your choice of mushrooms, chopped
- 1–2 tablespoons of pesto for each zucchini used
- 2–3 tablespoons of high-quality oil
- 1 teaspoon of dried rosemary
- 1 teaspoon of dried sage
- Chili flakes
- Sea salt and black pepper, to taste

INSTRUCTIONS

1. In a large bowl, lightly combine the meat, sea salt, pepper, rosemary, and sage.
2. Shape the mixture into meatballs and pan fry on medium-high heat in 1 tablespoon of oil until golden brown.
3. While the meatballs are cooking, spiralize your zucchini. Keep the skin on!
4. Remove the meatballs from the pan when done and add in another 1– 2 tablespoons of oil.
5. Add chopped mushrooms and cook for a few minutes before adding the spiralized noodles to the pan. Keep an eye on them, stirring and flipping them often. It only takes a couple of minutes. Remove from the heat when they begin to get golden brown.
6. On a plate, add a heaping tablespoon (or two) of your pesto to your zoodles and mushrooms, and mix in.
7. Add meatballs, and season with chili flakes.

TIPS

- If you are cooking for more than one person, pan-fry your zoodles only one zucchini at a time. If you try cooking two or more, they end up steaming instead of getting a little crispy. I like to add the pesto to the noodles after they are removed from the heat because pesto is raw and full of fresh nutrients and enzymes.

- If you're cooking with tomato sauce, you could add the sauce to the pan, and warm it up with the noodles.

- This recipe is equally delicious using shredded chicken instead of meatballs.

Beef Bolognese Sauce with Liver

INGREDIENTS

- 1 pound of medium ground, grass-fed beef
- 1 pound of lean ground, grass-fed beef
- 1 pound or less of grass-fed beef liver—to taste
- 1–3 cups of tomato sauce
- 2 tablespoons high-quality oil
- Pinch or two of sea salt

Optional: Chopped vegetables of your choosing.

INSTRUCTIONS

1. Add the medium and lean ground beef and salt, to a hot, well-oiled (large) pan.

2. Break the meat into smaller pieces using a spatula so that it is spread out across the pan.

3. While the meat starts to brown, put the liver into a food processor (or blender) and mix on high until smooth.

4. Add the liver to the pan when the ground beef is halfway cooked and browning.

5. Stir regularly to cook the beef mixture evenly.

6. Add the tomato sauce once the beef is almost cooked, and add in any extra, pre-cooked vegetables.

7. Continue to stir and simmer for about 5 minutes to evaporate some of the liquid and marinate the meat in the sauce.

Slow-Cooked Braised Beef Cheek Stew

Cooked in 48-Hour Bone Broth

Appropriately cooked, beef cheeks are so tender you can cut them with a spoon, and they are the perfect cut to make a rich, nutritious stew. Braising involves browning the beef on the pan, which helps bring out the flavor of the meat. It's not an essential step, and you could just put the raw beef cheeks into the broth if you're short on time, but braising adds some dimension to your stew.

This recipe is two in one. First, it calls for making bone broth and then using the broth to slow-cook your beef cheeks and turn it into a stew. By using broth that simmered for two days, you get all the nutritional benefits of bone broth plus the nutrients of the meat and vegetables.

You could purchase bone broth and use pre-made broth as a base for the stew or skip Steps 1 and 2 altogether and stew the beef cheek in regular water, not broth. Using broth makes the dish more flavorful and nutritious, but if you don't have the bones or the time, you can just put your cheeks in the slow cooker and let it simmer for 4–6 hours.

INGREDIENTS

- 1-1/2 pounds of beef cheeks
- 4 quarts of bone broth—enough to fill your slow cooker about 3/4 of the way.
- See *48-Hour Grass-Fed Beef Bone Marrow Broth* recipe for ingredients and instructions.
- 1/2 tablespoon dried rosemary
- 4-5 large carrots
- 1/2 large stalk of celery
- Sea salt and black pepper, to taste.

INSTRUCTIONS

1. Make your bone broth, and because the stew calls for adding carrots and celery, I opted not to include the carrots and celery in the broth. Feel free to leave out the vegetables from the broth portion of the recipe.

2. When your broth is ready, strain all the bones and return the broth into the slow cooker.

3. Sear your beef cheeks on a pan with high heat - brown the sides but leave the meat raw on the inside.

4. Add in your seared beef cheeks and rosemary, salt, and pepper, to the broth in the slow cooker. Let the cheeks simmer on high for 5-6 hours.

5. Add in the carrots and celery (chopped) to your stew and let simmer on low for about 30-45 minutes until the vegetables are tender.

TIPS

- It's important to use organic/pasture-raised/grass-fed bones for broth, for two reasons: First, bones store heavy metal contamination, so if your animal was exposed to GMO grain, and harmful chemicals during its life (unnatural feed/lifestyle), you will be extracting those stored neurotoxins and drinking a poisonous broth. Second, to get the benefits (amino profile, minerals), make sure the animal whose bones you're using have collected these nutrients over a lifetime which you are then extracting over a slow 48-hour simmer into your broth.

- Add the vegetables only at the very end of your simmer; otherwise, they will be complete mush by the time your meat is cooked.

- Feel free to play around with other cuts of stewing meats, and other vegetables.

- All the quantities for this recipe are completely up to you; basically, you want to fill your slow cooker 3/4 of the way with broth, then add in your stewing meat for 5-6 hours, and then add in your vegetables at the end to soften before serving.

48-Hour Grass-Fed Beef Bone Marrow Broth

INGREDIENTS

- 2–3 pounds of grass-fed beef bone-marrow bones
- 3 large carrots
- ½ large celery bunch
- A big knob of ginger
- 1 tablespoon rosemary
- Sea salt and black pepper, to taste
- A splash of apple cider vinegar
- 2–3 cloves of garlic (optional)

INSTRUCTIONS

1. Add ginger and garlic to a blender filled halfway with filtered water, and blend on high for 20 seconds.

2. Add the ginger/garlic water to your slow cooker and then continue to fill your slow cooker halfway with more filtered water.

3. Add a splash of apple cider vinegar.

4. Add the bones, carrots, celery, and seasonings.

5. Fill the slow cooker up with water until full.

6. Simmer on low for 48 hours.

7. After 48 hours (or up to 60 hours) strain the liquid discarding all the solids and store the liquid in a glass mason jar in the fridge for up to a week.

TIPS

- After about 24 hours, your broth will have evaporated a decent amount of liquid; refill the pot with more water.

- You can also freeze broth cubes to extend the life of the broth and keep it frozen.

- Your broth should be extremely fatty. Once cooled, you should notice a thick layer of fat on the top, which is a sign you made a quality broth. Do not discard this fat as it is nutrient-dense with use in other cooking. The broth should be opaque, golden, and full of vitamins and minerals.

Coconut Wraps

Coconut wraps are made of 100% coconut meat and make an excellent alternative to regular wheat-based wraps, and you can use them as you usually would a conventional breaded wrap.

IDEAS FOR COCONUT WRAPS

- Sardines, avocado, cucumber, and parsley with chili flakes, drizzled with olive oil.

- Tuna salad made with homemade mayo, celery, grated carrots, and pickles.

- Shredded chicken with lettuce, crispy oven-baked bacon, and avocado.

Roasted Leg of Lamb with Mint Yogurt

INGREDIENTS

- Leg of lamb (approximately 1-1/4 pounds)
- 3–4 pieces of garlic
- 1 bunch of fresh rosemary
- 2 tablespoons dried rosemary
- 1 tablespoon dried thyme
- Juice of half a lemon
- 1/4 cup olive oil
- Sea salt and black pepper, to taste

INSTRUCTIONS

1. Preheat the oven to 400° F.
2. Place minced garlic, herbs, juice of half a lemon, and about ¼ cup of olive oil in a bowl.
3. Rub all over the lamb and then season all over with salt and pepper.
4. Cook for 1 hour and 15 minutes for a pinker lamb, or 1 hour and 30 minutes for more well-done.

TIPS

- Whenever oven roasting meat, you can add your choice of vegetables in the pan to make a complete meal. Opt for lower-carb greens on a keto day (cabbage, broccoli) or starchier ones on a feast day (carrots, parsnips, sweet potato, pumpkin).

Ratatouille

INGREDIENTS

- 1 large eggplant
- 3 large tomatoes
- 2 red bell peppers
- 1 green bell pepper
- 2 large zucchinis
- 1 medium red onion
- 3 cloves of garlic
- 3 tablespoons olive oil
- ½ tablespoon dried oregano
- ¼ tablespoon dried thyme
- Sea salt and black pepper, to taste
- Fresh basil

INSTRUCTIONS

1. Put the oil, herbs, minced garlic, and finely diced onion in a large pot, over medium heat.

2. Once the onions have softened, add in all the other vegetables, roughly chopped.

3. Stir regularly while as the ratatouille starts cooking, but once the juices of the tomato have created somewhat of a stew, you can let the mix simmer on low heat (stirring occasionally). The longer it simmers, the more flavor will come out, even though it is complete after about 20 minutes of heat.

4. When cooked, top ratatouille with fresh basil, and another drizzle of olive oil.

Green Soup

INGREDIENTS

- 1 bunch of dandelion greens
- 1 bunch of celery
- 1 bunch of silverbeet or collard greens
- 1 large fennel bulb
- 1 bunch of parsley
- Knob of ginger
- Juice of half a lemon
- Sea salt and black pepper, to taste

INSTRUCTIONS

1. Fill a large pot halfway with filtered water, add all the ingredients, fill the rest of the pot with water, and turn the stove on high heat.

2. Once the water is boiling, turn down on low and let it simmer for about 10 minutes until the greens are soft, then turn off the heat.

3. Mix until smooth with a hand blender.

TIP

- Try blending ginger in a blender with a few cups of water instead of chopping it, and just adding the potent ginger-water to the soup mix (at the beginning, with the rest of the vegetables).

Chicken Zoodle Soup

INGREDIENTS

- 1/3 cup coconut oil or ghee
- 1 pound boneless, skinless chicken thighs or breasts, sliced (optional)
- 1 cup diced celery
- 2 shallots, diced
- 1/2 cup diced carrots
- 8 cups of chicken bone broth
- 2 teaspoons finely ground sea salt
- 1/2 teaspoon dried thyme
- 1 teaspoon dried or fresh parsley
- 2 cups baby spinach
- Fresh ground black pepper, to taste
- Spiralized zucchini noodles, or "Zoodles" (about 2-3 large zucchini, or 4-6 small)

INSTRUCTIONS

1. Heat the oil in a large saucepan over medium-high heat, then add the celery, shallots, and carrots to the pan and sauté for 5 minutes.
2. Add the broth, salt, thyme, parsley, and pepper. Cover and bring to a simmer.
3. Once simmering, reduce the heat to medium-low and cook for 20 minutes.
4. In the last 2 minutes of cooking, add the zoodles and the cooked, diced chicken (if using).
5. Put a small handful of chopped spinach in each bowl.
6. Remove from heat and divide the soup into the bowls, wilting the spinach.
7. Enjoy!

Cauliflower Crust Pizza

INGREDIENTS

- 1 large head of cauliflower (about 2–2.5 pounds of florets)
- 1 egg
- 1/3 cup soft goat cheese
- 1½ teaspoons dried oregano
- 1 teaspoon dried thyme
- Pinch of salt

INSTRUCTIONS

1. Preheat oven to 400° F.
2. Cut the cauliflower into florets and steam them until soft (about 5–7 minutes).
3. In a food processor, blend the cooked florets until you have a nice- looking texture—you might have to do this in batches depending on the size of your food processor.
4. This step is the key to a successful crust; strain the cauliflower rice. The only way to do this properly is to put the cauliflower in a cheesecloth (or dishcloth) and twist hard until the water comes out.
5. In a bowl, whisk the egg, and then add in all the rest of the ingredients.
6. Mix with your hands to form a dough. Shape the crust on a baking tray lined with parchment paper. This dough will not rise nor spread out like regular dough, so shape it thick enough to use as a crust (about 1/3" thick).
7. Bake for about 35 minutes until it becomes golden brown.
8. Remove from the oven, add your toppings, and bake again until toppings are melted and cooked to preference.

Nacho Salad

INGREDIENTS

- ½ pound of ground beef
- ½ red onion
- Tahini
- A handful of mushrooms
- 1 head of romaine lettuce
- 1 small tomato
- ½ an avocado
- 1 teaspoon rosemary
- 1 teaspoon thyme
- 1 spring onion, diced
- A pinch of cumin
- 1 tablespoon olive oil

Optional: Raw, cheddar cheese

INSTRUCTIONS

1. On an oiled pan, add onions, chopped mushrooms, ground beef, salt, pepper, rosemary, and thyme.

2. Stir until ground beef is cooked through (slightly browned).

3. Place the ground beef and mushroom mix on a bed of chopped lettuce and top with chopped tomatoes, avocado, a sprinkle of cumin, and diced spring onions.

Roast Chicken

A simple roast chicken is a staple recipe you should master. Roasting a whole chicken at a time will probably leave you with leftovers that you can easily use for lunch the next day.

INGREDIENTS

- 1 whole chicken
- 2-3 tablespoons of olive oil or butter
- 1 tablespoon rosemary
- 1 tablespoon thyme
- Sea salt and black pepper, to taste

INSTRUCTIONS

1. Preheat the oven to 350°F

2. On a baking tray, coat the entire chicken with olive oil, or melted butter. Rub the herbs on to cover it all over with black pepper and sea salt to taste.

3. Cook in the oven on the middle rack for approximately 40 minutes. Cooking time will depend on the size of the chicken. It is done when the outside skin is golden brown and crisp.

TIP

- To ensure a juicy, golden brown roast chicken, baste the chicken in its juices a couple of times throughout the cook; it will prevent the skin from burning and allow it to retain more moisture.

Beef Liver Pâté

INGREDIENTS

- ½ pound of grass-fed, beef liver
- 1 small onion, any variety, finely diced
- 1/3 cup + 2 tablespoons beef tallow, OR butter, OR ghee
- 1 tablespoon rosemary
- A pinch of sage
- Sea salt, black pepper, to taste

INSTRUCTIONS

1. Heat a large frying pan, add 2 tablespoons olive oil and sauté finely diced onions, rosemary, sage, pepper, and sea salt.
2. Stir until onions are golden brown and then add in the beef liver.
3. Once the liver is cooked through, cool, and place all the ingredients in a food processor.
4. Add in the rest of the fat (1/3 cup) and then blend until the pâté is smooth and creamy.

KETOSIS-FRIENDLY RECIPES LOW CARBOHYDRATE
SIDES AND SAUCES

Activated Walnut and Wild Rocket Pesto

This pesto is full of real, whole foods and is a perfect way to incorporate more fat into your diet. You can put it on anything from cauliflower pizza to zucchini noodles, oven-roasted squash, oven-baked chicken or even use it as a dip for sweet potato fries. The recipe calls for "activated nuts," which means nuts that were soaked, and dehydrated. You can easily make your own, buy them activated, or use soaked nuts without dehydrating them or use regular raw or roasted nuts.

INGREDIENTS

- 4 cups basil
- 4 cups wild rocket arugula
- 1 cup olive oil
- ½ cup walnuts
- 3–4 cloves garlic
- A squeeze of fresh lemon juice
- Sea salt and black pepper, to taste

INSTRUCTIONS

1. Mix all ingredients, except olive oil, in a food processor until well chopped.
2. Slowly add in the olive oil and continue to blend until smooth.

Classic Greek Salad

INGREDIENTS

- 2 tomatoes, chopped
- 1/2 of a large cucumber, chopped
- 4 tablespoons olive oil
- 1/2 cup of feta, crumbled
- A handful of olives
- 1 teaspoon of wild oregano
- Salt and pepper, to taste

Optional: Capers, to taste

INSTRUCTIONS

1. Mix all ingredients in a bowl! Ideally, let sit in the fridge for 30-60 minutes before serving.

Shaved Zucchini and Fennel Salad

INGREDIENTS

- 2 pounds zucchini
- ½ a bulb fennel
- *1/3* cup olive oil
- Juice of half a lemon
- Pinch of sea salt
- Pinch of black pepper
- Pinch of dried rosemary
- A handful of toasted hazelnuts, crushed

INSTRUCTIONS

1. Prepare the dressing. Whisk oil, lemon juice, sea salt, black pepper, and rosemary, and set aside.
2. Using a mandolin slicer or thick peeler, peel the zucchini into ribbons.
3. Using a mandolin slicer or a sharp knife, shave the fennel into thin slices.
4. Toss the zucchini and fennel in the dressing and top with crushed toasted hazelnuts.

Garlic Green Beans

INGREDIENTS

- 1 pound green beans
- 2-3 cloves garlic
- 3 tablespoons olive oil, ghee, or butter
- Sea salt and black pepper, to taste

INSTRUCTIONS

1. In a pan brown minced garlic and oil/butter, on medium heat.
2. Once the garlic browns, add in green beans and toss until beans begin to char.
3. Remove from heat, and season to taste.

Spicy Turmeric Roasted Cauliflower

INGREDIENTS

- 1 head of cauliflower
- 1 tablespoon turmeric powder
- 1 teaspoon paprika
- Sea salt and black pepper, to taste
- Olive oil or butter to cover the whole cauliflower

Optional: Pinch of cayenne pepper

INSTRUCTIONS

1. Preheat the oven to 400° F.
2. Coat the cauliflower pieces with oil or melted butter in a bowl, then add spices.
3. Spread cauliflower evenly on a lightly oiled tray.
4. Bake 30-45 minutes until the cauliflower turns golden brown.

Cauliflower Mash

INGREDIENTS

- 1 large cauliflower, chopped
- Olive Oil
- 3-4 tablespoons of ghee or butter
- 1 sprig of spring onion
- Sea salt and black pepper, to taste

INSTRUCTIONS

1. Preheat the oven to 400°F
2. Coat chopped up cauliflower florets in olive oil and roast until golden brown—about 35 minutes.
3. Put roasted cauliflower, butter, and spring onion, salt, and pepper in the food processor and blend until smooth.

Avocado Gazpacho

INGREDIENTS

- 4 large ripe avocados
- 3 large cucumbers
- 2 large tomatoes
- 1/2 red onion
- 1 bunch cilantro
- 2 cloves garlic
- 2 cups filtered water, or bone broth (chilled)
- 1 tablespoon olive oil
- Juice one lime
- Sea salt and black pepper, to taste

INSTRUCTIONS

1. Add all the ingredients into a high-powered blender and blend until smooth.
2. Either refrigerate and serve chilled or add in a few ice cubes and blend again, until smooth and serve straight away.

Guacamole

INGREDIENTS

- 2-3 large avocados
- 1 teaspoon of cumin powder
- 1/4 red onion, finely chopped
- A squeeze of fresh lemon or lime juice, or a few tablespoons of sauerkraut juice
- Sea salt and pepper, to taste

INSTRUCTIONS

1. Mix all the ingredients in a bowl.

TIP

- Serve guacamole chilled. Turn the guacamole into a complete meal by mashing in a can of your preferred fish—sardines, mackerel, tuna, or anchovies, or add chopped tomatoes, and use as a dip with carrots!

Lemon Tahini Sauce

INGREDIENTS

- ½ cup tahini
- 2/3 cup of filtered water
- Juice of one whole lemon
- A handful of fresh parsley, chopped
- 2 tablespoons olive oil
- 1 clove of garlic, minced
- Sea salt and black pepper, to taste

INSTRUCTIONS

1. Put all the ingredients into a food processor and process on high until smooth. You may need to add a little more water depending on the desired consistency.

Spicy Oven-Roasted Cashews

INGREDIENTS

- 2 pounds raw cashews
- 2 teaspoons paprika
- Juice of 1/2 lime
- 2 tablespoons olive oil
- 1 teaspoon cayenne pepper
- 1 teaspoon cumin
- 1 teaspoon of sea salt
- Black pepper, to taste

INSTRUCTIONS

1. Preheat the oven to 400° F.
2. Place all the ingredients in a bowl and toss to coat evenly.
3. Place the cashews spread out evenly on a baking tray lined with parchment paper.
4. Roast in the oven until golden brown, approximately 20 minutes, turning halfway.

KETOSIS-FRIENDLY RECIPES LOW CARBOHYDRATE
DESSERTS

Chocolate Collagen Almond Butter Cups

INGREDIENTS

- ¼ cup of coconut oil
- ½ cup cacao butter
- ½ cup coconut butter
- ¼ cup collagen powder
- 1 cup cold pressed raw cacao
- ¼ cup almond butter
- Pinch of sea salt
- Pinch of cinnamon
- A silicon mold in which to make your chocolates, or an ice cube tray

INSTRUCTIONS

1. Melt the coconut oil, cacao butter, and coconut butter in a double boiler, then take off the stove.

2. Whisk in cacao, collagen, salt, and cinnamon, until smooth.

3. Fill half the mold with chocolate, add a dollop of almond butter, then fill the rest of the mold with chocolate.

4. Freeze for at least 15 minutes before consuming, and store in the fridge or freezer.

5. Making your chocolate is a surprisingly easy way to nourish your body and up your dose of healthy fats. This recipe has no added sugar, and you can interchange whatever nut butter you like for the filling.

Collagen Cookie Dough Balls

INGREDIENTS

Dry Ingredients:

- ¾ cup brazil nuts
- ½ cup walnuts
- ¼ cup pumpkin seeds
- ¼ cup cashews
- 2 teaspoons chia seeds
- 1 cup shredded coconut
- ¼ cup of collagen powder
- 2 tablespoons cacao nibs, or to taste
- 2½ tablespoons cacao powder
- 2 tablespoons raw maca powder
- 1 teaspoon cinnamon powder
- ½ teaspoon vanilla bean powder
- Pinch of sea salt

Wet Ingredients:

- ½ cup coconut butter, melted
- ¼ cup coconut oil, melted
- A splash of coconut or almond milk

Optional: Two to three large dates

INSTRUCTIONS

1. For crunchier balls, put all the dry ingredients *except cacao, and cacao nibs* in a food processor and pulse; for smoother, blend well.

2. Add liquids, and process again until a dough forms.

3. Note: You may not need the nut milk at all. Try blending first to see the consistency and add nut milk if needed.

4. Add in cacao nibs and pulse just a few times or mix them in by hand.

5. Roll into balls of whatever size you prefer.

6. Note: If you want to make ½ of the batch double chocolate, at this point remove ½ the "batter" and then add in the cacao powder, blend again, and you'll have ½ regular cookie dough, and ½ double chocolate. If you want the entire batch to be double chocolate, add in the cacao powder in Step 1.

7. Store in the fridge or the freezer and thaw for 5–10 minutes before consuming.

TIPS

- You may substitute any nuts in this recipe or use seeds if preferred. Cashews and almonds also work well.

Chocolate Hazelnut Spread

INGREDIENTS

- 1½ cups of toasted hazelnuts
- 4 tablespoons of cacao powder
- 1 tablespoon of coconut oil, melted
- ¼ cup coconut butter, melted
- 1 teaspoon vanilla powder or extract
- Pinch of sea salt

Optional: One to two tablespoons of honey or monk fruit extract

INSTRUCTIONS

1. Blend hazelnuts in a food processor on high until finely ground.
2. Add in the melted oil and coconut butter while the food processor is still on high.
3. Add in remaining ingredients and process on high until smooth paste forms.
4. Store in the refrigerator.

FEAST DAY FRIENDLY RECIPES (HIGHER CARBOHYDRATE)

Note: Feast (higher carbohydrate) days do not mean unhealthy days. Carbohydrates play a crucial role in creating metabolic flexibility in the body and ensuring you continue to progress along your health journey.

Ideally, you would take a recipe from the low-carb list and add some higher carbohydrate vegetables and fruits with natural sugars, such as like sweet potato, squash. In fact, the "desserts" are so nutrient-dense you could truly have them for breakfast!

FEAST DAY-FRIENDLY RECIPES
HIGH CARBOHYDRATE
BREAKFAST

Sweet Potato Almond Butter Smoothie

INGREDIENTS

- 1 cup of sweet potato, previously baked
- A handful of toasted coconut flakes
- ¼ cup almond milk
- 1 cup of filtered water
- 2 tablespoons almond butter
- 1 teaspoon cinnamon
- 1 teaspoon nutmeg powder

Optional: One scoop of collagen powder or protein powder

INSTRUCTIONS

1. Place all the ingredients in a blender and blend on high until smooth and creamy.

Super Green Smoothie with Banana

INGREDIENTS

- 1 banana, frozen
- 1/3 avocado, frozen
- ¼ cup fennel
- A handful of greens of your choice - spinach, kale, arugula, or a combination
- A handful of fresh mint
- ½ cup cucumber
- ½ cup full-fat coconut milk
- 2 cups of filtered water

Optional: One teaspoon chlorella powder

Optional: One scoop of collagen powder or protein powder

INSTRUCTIONS

1. Place all the ingredients in a blender and blend on high until smooth.

Caramel Smoothie with Dates

INGREDIENTS

- 1 banana, frozen
- 2 tablespoons cashew butter
- 2 dates
- 1 tablespoon tahini
- 1 teaspoon maca powder
- 1 cup ice

Optional: One scoop of collagen powder or protein powder

INSTRUCTIONS

1. Place all the ingredients in a blender and blend on high until smooth.

Chia Matcha Delight Smoothie

INGREDIENTS

- 1 cup yogurt of choice
- 1 tablespoon raw honey
- 1 teaspoon matcha powder
- 1 tablespoon coconut oil
- 2 tablespoons chia seeds (soaked in 8 tbsp of water for at least 20 minutes)
- 1/2 to 1 cup ice cubes
- Pinch sea salt

Optional: 1 cup steamed kale

Optional: 1 raw, pastured egg

INSTRUCTIONS

1. Put ice cubes in bottom of the blender first and then add in the rest of the ingredients and blend on high.

Lettuce Detox Smoothie

INGREDIENTS

- 4 cups of filtered water
- 2 cups romaine lettuce
- 2 tablespoons fresh parsley
- 1 tablespoon fresh ginger, peeled and chopped
- 1 cup of cucumber, sliced
- 1 kiwi fruit, chopped (skin on)
- 1 avocado (remove pit and scoop the flesh out of shell)
- 1 tablespoon raw honey
- Pinch sea salt

Optional: 1 teaspoon spirulina

Optional: 1 cup of chopped celery

INSTRUCTIONS

1. Put ice cubes in bottom of the blender first, and then add in the rest of the ingredients and blend on high.

Nutty Green Smoothie

INGREDIENTS

- 16 ounces chilled, tea of choice
- 1 can full-fat coconut milk
- 2-4 cups raw spinach
- 1/2 cup raw cashews
- 1/4 cup chia seeds
- 1/2 teaspoon turmeric
- 1/2 teaspoon cinnamon
- 1/2 tablespoon raw honey
- 1 cup of ice cubes
- Pinch sea salt

INSTRUCTIONS

1. Put ice cubes in bottom of the blender first, and then add in the rest of the ingredients and blend on high.

Cocoa Pumpkin Pudding Smoothie

INGREDIENTS

- 1/2 can pumpkin puree
- 1/2 can unsweetened, full-fat coconut milk
- 2 tablespoons gelatin powder
- 4 tablespoons cup cocoa powder
- 1 teaspoon pumpkin pie spice
- Pinch sea salt
- 1 tablespoon raw honey to taste (optional)

INSTRUCTIONS

1. Put all ingredients, excluding gelatin, in a high-speed blender and mix on high speed.

2. Once thoroughly mixed, add gelatin and incorporate at low speed.

Carrot Cake Shake

INGREDIENTS

- 1 can unsweetened, full-fat coconut milk
- 2-3 medium carrots, chopped
- 1 avocado
- 1 frozen banana
- 2 tablespoons collagen powder
- 2 tablespoons gelatin powder
- 1 teaspoon cinnamon
- 1 teaspoon ginger
- 1 small scoop raisins (optional)

INSTRUCTIONS

1. Put all ingredients, excluding collagen and gelatin, in a high-speed blender and mix on high speed.

2. Once thoroughly mixed, add collagen and gelatin and incorporate at low speeds.

Ruby Red Zinger Smoothie

INGREDIENTS

- 1 can unsweetened, full-fat coconut milk
- 2 small beets, scrubbed and chopped
- 1 orange, peeled
- 2 large carrots, chopped
- 1-inch piece fresh ginger or 1 teaspoon of ginger powder
- 1 teaspoon turmeric powder
- 2 tablespoons collagen
- 1 teaspoon of sea salt

INSTRUCTIONS

1. Put all ingredients, excluding collagen, in a high-speed blender and mix on high speed. Once thoroughly mixed, add collagen and incorporate at low speed.

Banana Pancakes with Homemade Coconut Yogurt and Cinnamon

INGREDIENTS

- 1 large banana (ripe)
- 2 eggs
- Pinch aluminum free baking powder
- 1/2 teaspoon vanilla powder or extract
- Pinch sea salt
- Dollop Homemade Coconut Yogurt
- Dash Ceylon cinnamon
- Coconut oil

INSTRUCTIONS

1. Mash the banana with a fork until smooth, and then mix in the eggs, baking powder, vanilla, and salt.

2. Cook on medium heat on a well coconut-oiled pan until golden brown.

3. Top with Homemade Coconut Yogurt and a dash of cinnamon.

Sweet Breakfast Muffins

INGREDIENTS

- 2 cups almond flour
- 2 teaspoons baking soda
- 1 teaspoon Ceylon cinnamon
- Pinch sea salt
- 1/2 cup very ripe banana (mashed)
- 1/3 cup sweet potato (roasted)
- 1 egg
- 4 tablespoons coconut oil
- 1 tablespoon vanilla powder or extract
- 1 tablespoon fresh lemon juice
- 1/2 cup walnuts (chopped)
- 1/2 cup coconut flakes

INSTRUCTIONS

1. Preheat the oven to 350°F.
2. In a large bowl, mix the almond flour, baking soda, Ceylon cinnamon, and salt.
3. In a separate bowl, mix the banana, sweet potato egg, coconut oil, vanilla, and lemon juice until smooth.
4. Gently mix the dry and wet ingredients.
5. Add in the walnuts and coconut.
6. Fill paper-lined muffin tins 3/4 the way to the top and bake for approximately 20-22 minutes, until golden brown.
7. Cool before serving.

FEAST DAY-FRIENDLY RECIPES
HIGH CARBOHYDRATE
LUNCH AND DINNER

Sweet Potato "Toast"

Sweet potato can be an incredible alternative to a slice of bread when done properly. The sweetness of the vegetable makes for a great platform for toppings, and much more nutritious meal.

INGREDIENTS

- 1 large sweet potato
- 1 teaspoon olive oil
- Your choice of toppings

INSTRUCTIONS

1. Slice sweet potato in lengths, about 1/3 inch thick.
2. Brush both sides with olive oil.
3. Either roast in the oven on a baking tray lined with parchment paper (at 400°F for 20 minutes, flipping halfway through) or use a conventional toaster and continue to toast until sides are golden brown (it will take a few times).
4. Top with your choice of sweet or savory toppings!

IDEAS FOR SWEET POTATO TOAST TOPPINGS

- Avocado, smoked salmon, chives, and sea salt
- Almond butter, raspberry jam, blueberries, and cacao nibs
- Cottage cheese, wild honey, and cinnamon

Lentils and Warm Vegetable Stir-Fry with Olives and Basil

INGREDIENTS

- 2 cups of French green lentils
- 1 red pepper
- 1 large zucchini
- 1 medium eggplant
- 1 large tomato
- ½ tablespoons dried oregano powder
- 2 teaspoons dried thyme
- 1 teaspoon of sea salt
- 1 teaspoon black pepper
- Olive oil
- Fresh basil
- Handful of olives

INSTRUCTIONS

1. Bring water to a simmer and cook lentils until soft (about 15-20 minutes).

2. Meanwhile, add all the rest of the vegetable, chopped, to a large pan with a generous amount of olive oil, thyme, oregano, salt, and pepper.

3. Stir vegetables until thoroughly cooked.

4. Strain lentils and put on a plate, top with vegetable stir-fry, chopped fresh basil, a drizzle of olive oil, and a handful of olives.

Carrot Soup Drizzled with Olive Oil and Prosciutto

Carrots are an all right vegetable in moderation on a ketogenic day, but as a soup, it will probably tip you over into a feast day meal. Combine it with some extra fat and a small portion of protein, and you have yourself a delicious meal.

INGREDIENTS

- 6 large carrots
- 3 parsnips
- 1 large onion
- 4 cloves of garlic, whole
- 4 large tomatoes
- 4 tablespoons olive oil
- Juice of half a lemon
- A handful of fresh basil
- 1 teaspoon cumin powder
- Sea salt and black pepper, to taste

Optional: One to two cups of bone broth

INSTRUCTIONS

1. Preheat oven to 400° F.

2. On a baking tray, roast carrots, parsnips, garlic, onions, and to-matoes, coated generously in olive oil, salt, pepper, and cumin (30-35 minutes, tossing halfway through).

3. In a high-speed blender, blend the roasted vegetables with the rest of the ingredients until smooth. You can add in filtered water or bone broth to achieve desired consistency.

4. Top the soup with fresh basil.

FEAST DAY-FRIENDLY RECIPES
HIGH CARBOHYDRATE
SIDES AND SAUCES

Crispy Sweet Potato Fries

INGREDIENTS

- Sweet potatoes—whatever quantity
- High-quality oil of your choice
- Sea salt to taste

Optional: Dried rosemary

INSTRUCTIONS

1. Preheat oven to 400 °F.
2. Chop sweet potato into preferred size wedges with the skin.
3. In a bowl, drizzle a small amount of oil on the wedges, and cover the fries evenly. Add in a tablespoon of dried rosemary if desired and toss throughout the fries.
4. Lay out the fries on a baking tray lined with parchment paper, leaving space between each fry.
5. Bake for 15 minutes, then flip the fries and bake another 15 minutes. Depending on how your oven cooks leave them in until they are golden and crispy on the outside.

TIPS

- Don't use too much oil; coat them very lightly, they shouldn't be dripping in oil.
- If the fries are touching or you try to jam too many on the tray, your sweet potatoes will steam instead of bake. When I make big batches, I use two trays.
- If you're only baking one tray of sweet potato, cook the fries on one of the highest racks from the oven. If baking more than one, use a high rack, and the rack just below the upper tray. There is something about doing it that way that just works.

Sweet Potato Mash

INGREDIENTS

- 2-3 large sweet potatoes
- 4 tablespoons of ghee or butter
- 1 teaspoon of Ceylon cinnamon
- Sea salt and black pepper, to taste

INSTRUCTIONS

1. Chop sweet potato and steam or oven roast until cooked. Steaming is faster, roasting is more flavorful.
2. In a pot, add sweet potato, butter, cinnamon, salt, and pepper and mash until smooth.

Roasted Vegetables Drizzled with Olive Oil and Sea Salt

Every vegetable is delicious when roasted, from carrots and sweet potatoes, to parsnips, peppers, asparagus, cauliflower, and broccoli. More water-based vegetables (like zucchini or asparagus) will roast faster than starchier ones (like potatoes) so pair similar vegetables while you cook them or toss in the quicker-to-roast ones in towards the end.

INGREDIENTS

- 1 large zucchini
- 2 large red peppers
- A handful of mushrooms
- 4 large carrots
- 4 parsnips
- A hefty drizzle of olive oil, tallow, or butter
- 1 tablespoon rosemary
- 1/2 tablespoon thyme
- Sea salt and black pepper, to taste

INSTRUCTIONS

1. Preheat the oven to 400°F.
2. Leaving the skin on, roughly chop all the vegetables.
3. On a baking tray, cover the vegetables with a decent amount of olive oil, the herbs, salt, and pepper, and mix with your hands to evenly coat.
4. Spread out vegetables so that they are even across the pan and bake for approximately 40 minutes, giving the vegetables a good toss halfway through.

Hasselback Potatoes

INGREDIENTS

- 4 potatoes (or sweet potatoes)
- A drizzle of olive oil per potato (or melted butter)
- Sea salt to taste

Optional: A dollop of fresh sour cream, and chives

INSTRUCTIONS

1. Preheat the oven to 400°F.

2. Finely cut the entire length of the potato, leaving about 1/2 a cm from the bottom (don't cut the slices completely through).

3. On a pan, spread out the potatoes, drizzle them with oil or melted butter.

4. Roast until golden brown—time will depend on the size of the potato, about 40 minutes.

FEAST DAY-FRIENDLY RECIPES
HIGH CARBOHYDRATE
DESSERTS

Sweet Potato Brownies

INGREDIENTS

- 2-1/2 cups sweet potato, roasted and mashed
- 3 eggs
- 1/4 cup almond butter
- 1/3 cup coconut oil
- 3/4 cup ground walnuts (or nut of your choice)
- 4 tablespoons pure maple syrup
- 8 dates
- 1/3 cup cacao or cocoa powder
- 1 teaspoon baking powder
- Pinch of salt

INSTRUCTIONS

1. Preheat oven to 350°F.
2. Mix all dry ingredients in a bowl and mix all wet ingredients in a separate bowl.
3. Combine wet and dry ingredients, whisk well.
4. Pour batter into a well-greased pan and bake for approximately 30 minutes (until a toothpick comes out clean).

Keto Lemon Cheesecake Bars
with Blueberry Sauce

INGREDIENTS

Crust:

- 2 large eggs
- 1 1/2 cups almond flour
- 1/2 Tbsp. cinnamon
- 1/4 cup xylitol
- 1/3 cup butter, melted
- 1/2 tsp. sea salt
- 1/2 tsp. baking powder

Cheesecake filling:

- 3 packages full-fat, organic cream cheese
- 3 large eggs
- 1/2 cup xylitol
- 1 tsp. vanilla
- 1/2 tsp. sea salt
- 4 Tbsp. fresh lemon juice
- 8-10 drops lemon essential oil (suggestion: doTerra)
- Garnish: organic lemon zest

Blueberry topping (optional):

- One 10oz. bag frozen blueberries
- 2 tablespoons xylitol
- 2 tablespoons arrowroot

INSTRUCTIONS

For crust:

1. Preheat oven to 325° F.

2. Mix all ingredients together. Add more butter or coconut oil if too dry.

3. Evenly distribute crust mixture into a 9" x 13" pan.

4. Bake crust for 18-20 minutes.

For cheesecake, topping and assembly:

1. While crust is baking, place all filling ingredients in large mixing bowl and combine with hand mixer until fully incorporated.

2. Once crust is lightly browned, remove from oven (leave oven on).

3. Spread cheesecake mixture evening over crust.

4. Garnish with lemon zest.

5. Bake cheesecake at 325° F for 45 minutes.

6. Make topping: put blueberries, xylitol and arrowroot in sauce-pan and heat over medium. Stir intermittently until warm and gooey.

7. Once down, allow to cool and then set in fridge for 1-2 hours, or until firm.

8. Slice into bars. Top with blueberry sauce and a sprinkle of sea salt.

9. Enjoy!

Variation without crust:

1. Make filling and pour into ramekins.

2. Bake at 325° F for 45 minutes.

3. Top with blueberry sauce and enjoy.

Salted Peanut Butter Bites

INGREDIENTS

- 1/2 cup unsweetened peanut butter or other nut or seed butter

- 1/4 cup coconut butter, melted – To melt coconut butter, place it in a small saucepan over low heat and stir constantly until it's fully melted

- 2 scoops grass-fed collagen peptides

- 1/4 tsp. pure vanilla extract

- 2 pinches ground cinnamon

- 2 pinches sea salt

- 8-10 drops stevia extract

- Extra salt for topping, if desired (this is highly recommended)

INSTRUCTIONS

1. Mix all the ingredients together until well combined. I recommend using a glass measuring cup with a spout for easy pouring.

2. Taste and add more stevia or salt, if desired.

3. Pour the mixture evenly into molds or mini cupcake liners, and sprinkle with a little extra salt

4. Place in the refrigerator until completely chilled and set, about 30 minutes.

ENDNOTES

Introduction

1. Prolonged fasting reduces IGF-1/PKA to promote hematopoietic-stem-cell-based regeneration and reverse immunosuppression. Cell Stem Cell. 2014 Jun 5;14(6):810-23. DOI: 10.1016/j.stem.2014.04.014. Cheng CW, Adams GB, Perin L, Wei M, Zhou X, Lam BS, Da Sacco S, Mirisola M, Quinn DI, Dorff TB, Kopchick JJ, Longo VD.

Chapter 1

1. Ketogenic diet attenuates neuronal injury via autophagy and mitochondrial pathways in pentylenetetrazol-kindled seizures. Bao- Hui Wang, Qun Hou, Yu-Qiang Lu, Meng-meng JIA, Tao Qiu, Xiao-hang Wang, Zheng-Xiang Zhang, Yan Jiang DOI:10.1016/j.brainres.2017.10.009.

2. Nutritional Ketosis and Mitohormesis: Potential Implications for Mitochondrial Function and Human. Health Journal of Nutrition and Metabolism. Volume 2018, Article ID 5157645, 27 pages https://DOI.org/10.1155/2018/5157645 , Vincent J. Miller, Frederick A. Villamena, and Jeff S. Volek.

3. Autophagy in stem cells. Autophagy. 2013 Jun 1; 9(6): 830–849. published online 2013 Mar 13. DOI: [10.4161/auto.24132]PMCID: PMC3672294 PMID: 23486312. Jun-Lin Guan, Anna Katharina Simon, Mark Prescott, Javier A. Menendez, Fei Liu, Fen Wang, Chenran Wang, Ernst Wolvetang, Alejandro Vazquez-Martin, and Jue Zhang.

4. Therapeutic ketosis with ketone ester delays central nervous system oxygen toxicity seizures in rats. Obesity, Diabetes and Energy Homeostasis. 15 May 2013 https://DOI.org/10.1152/ aj-pregu.00506.2012. Dominic P. D'Agostino, Raffaele Pilla, Heather E. Held, Carol S. Landon, Michelle Puchowicz, Henri Brunengraber, Csilla Ari, Patrick Arnold, and Jay B. Dean.

5. Rate of early onset Alzheimer's disease: a systematic review and meta-analysis. Ann Transl Med. 2015 Mar; 3(3): 38. DOI: [10.3978/j.issn.2305-5839.2015.01.19] PMCID: PMC4356853 PMID:25815299. Xi-Chen Zhu, Lan Tan, Hui-Fu Wang, Teng Jiang, Lei Cao, Chong Wang, Jun Wang, Chen-Chen Tan, Xiang-Fei Meng, and Jin-Tai Yu corresponding author.

6. Ketogenic diet for treatment of intractable epilepsy in adults: A meta-analysis of observational studies. Epilepsia Open. 2018 Feb 19;3(1):9-17. DOI: 10.1002/epi4.12098. eCollection 2018 Mar. Liu H, Yang Y, Wang Y, Tang H, Zhang F, Zhang Y, Zhao Y.

7. The ketogenic diet reverses gene expression patterns and reduces reactive oxygen species levels when used as an adjuvant therapy for glioma. *Nutr Metab (Lond).* 2010 Sep 10;7:74. doi: 10.1186/1743-7075-7-74. Stafford P1, Abdelwahab MG, Kim DY, Preul MC, Rho JM, Scheck AC.

8. The therapeutic implications of ketone bodies: the effects of ketone bodies in pathological conditions: ketosis, ketogenic diet, redox states, insulin resistance, and mitochondrial metabolism. *Prostaglandins Leukot Essent Fatty Acids.* 2004 Mar;70(3):309-19. Veech RL.

9. Ibid.

10. Ibid.

11. Ibid.

12. Ibid.

13. Ibid.

14. Ketogenic diets, mitochondria, and neurological diseases. *J Lipid Res.* 2014 Nov;55(11):2211-28. DOI: 10.1194/jlr.R048975. Epub 2014 May 20. Gano LB, Patel M, Rho JM.

15. Very-low-carbohydrate ketogenic diet v. low-fat diet for long-term weight loss: a meta-analysis of randomized controlled trials. *Br J Nutr.* 2013 Oct;110(7):1178-87. DOI: 10.1017/S0007114513000548. Epub 2013 May 7. Bueno NB, de Melo IS, de Oliveira SL, da Rocha Ataide T.

16. The ketogenic diet for type II bipolar disorder. *Neurocase.* 2013;19(5):423-6. DOI: 10.1080/13554794.2012.690421. Epub 2012 Oct 3. Phelps JR, Siemers SV, El-Mallakh RS.

17. The therapeutic implications of ketone bodies: the effects of ketone bodies in pathological conditions: ketosis, ketogenic diet, redox states, insulin resistance, and mitochondrial metabolism. *Prostaglandins Leukot Essent Fatty Acids.* 2004 Mar;70(3):309-19. Veech RL.

18. Ibid.

19. Ibid.

20. Ketogenic diet enhances neurovascular function with altered gut microbiome in young healthy mice *Sci Rep.* 2018; 8: 6670. Published online 2018 Apr 27. DOI: [10.1038/s41598-018-25190-5] PMCID: PMC5923270 PMID: 29703936 David Ma, Amy C. Wang, Ishita Parikh, Stefan J. Green, Jared D. Hoffman, George Chlipala, M. Paul Murphy, Brent S. Sokola, Björn Bauer, Anika M. S. Hartz, and Ai-Ling Lin.

21. The therapeutic implications of ketone bodies: the effects of ketone bodies in pathological conditions: ketosis, ketogenic diet, redox states, insulin resistance, and mitochondrial metabolism. *Prostaglandins Leukot Essent Fatty Acids.* 2004 Mar;70(3):309-19. Veech RL.

22. Ibid.

23. Ibid.

24. Ibid.

25. The Effects of Ketogenic Diet on Seizures, Cognitive Functions, and Other Neurological Disorders in Classical Phenotype of Glucose Transporter 1 Deficiency Syndrome. *Neuropediatrics.* 2015 Oct;46(5):313-20. DOI: 10.1055/s-0035-1558435. Epub 2015 Aug 12. Gumus H, Bayram AK, Kardas F, Canpolat M, Çağlayan AO, Kumandas S, Kendirci M.

26. THE NEUROPROTECTIVE PROPERTIES OF CALORIE RESTRICTION, THE KETOGENIC DIET, AND KETONE BODIES. *Brain*

Res Rev. 2009 Mar; 59(2): 293–315. Published online 2008 Sep 25. DOI: [10.1016/j.brainresrev.2008.09.002] PMCID: PMC2649682 NIHMSID: NIHMS75902 PMID: 18845187 Marwan A. Maalouf, Jong M. Rho, and Mark P. Mattson.

27. Very-low-carbohydrate ketogenic diet v. low-fat diet for long-term weight loss: a meta-analysis of randomized controlled trials. *Br J Nutr.* 2013 Oct;110(7):1178-87. DOI: 10.1017/S0007114513000548. Epub 2013 May 7. Bueno NB, de Melo IS, de Oliveira SL, da Rocha Ataide T.

28. The Effects of Ketogenic Diet on Seizures, Cognitive Functions, and Other Neurological Disorders in Classical Phenotype of Glucose Transporter 1 Deficiency Syndrome. *europediatrics.* 2015 Oct;46(5):313-20. DOI: 10.1055/s-0035-1558435. Epub 2015 Aug 12. Gumus H, Bayram AK, Kardas F, Canpolat M, Çağlayan AO, Kumandas S, Kendirci M, Per H.

29. Ibid.

30. Ibid.

31. Ketogenic Diet and Other Dietary Intervention Strategies in the Treatment of Cancer. *Curr Med Chem.* 2017;24(12):1170-1185. DOI: 10.2174/0929867324666170116122915. Vergati M, Krasniqi E, Monte GD, Riondino S, Vallone D, Guadagni F, Ferroni P, Roselli M.

32. Nutrition and acne: therapeutic potential of ketogenic diets. *Skin Pharmacol Physiol.* 2012;25(3):111-7. DOI: 10.1159/000336404. Epub 2012 Feb 11. Paoli A, Grimaldi K, Toniolo L, Canato M, Bianco A, Fratter A.

33. The effects of a low-carbohydrate, ketogenic diet on the polycystic ovary syndrome: A pilot study *Nutr Metab* (Lond). 2005; 2: 35. Published online 2005 Dec 16. DOI: [10.1186/1743-7075-2-35] PMCID: PMC1334192 PMID: 16359551 John C Mavropoulos, William S Yancy, Juanita Hepburn, and Eric C Westman.

34. The therapeutic implications of ketone bodies: the effects of ketone bodies in pathological conditions: ketosis, ketogenic diet, redox states, insulin resistance, and mitochondrial metabolism.

Prostaglandins Leukot Essent Fatty Acids. 2004 Mar;70(3):309-19. Veech RL.

35. The Effects of Ketogenic Diet on Seizures, Cognitive Functions, and Other Neurological Disorders in Classical Phenotype of Glucose Transporter 1 Deficiency Syndrome. *Europediatrics.* 2015 Oct;46(5):313-20. DOI: 10.1055/s-0035-1558435. Epub 2015 Aug 12. Gumus H, Bayram AK, Kardas F, Canpolat M, Çağlayan AO, Kumandas S, Kendirci M, Per H.

36. The therapeutic implications of ketone bodies: the effects of ketone bodies in pathological conditions: ketosis, ketogenic diet, redox states, insulin resistance, and mitochondrial metabolism. *Prostaglandins Leukot Essent Fatty Acids.* 2004 Mar;70(3):309-19. Veech RL.

37. Ibid.

38. Ketogenic diet enhances neurovascular function with altered gut microbiome in young healthy mice *Sci Rep.* 2018; 8: 6670. Published online 2018 Apr 27. DOI: [10.1038/s41598-018-25190-5] PMCID: PMC5923270 PMID: 29703936 David Ma, Amy C. Wang, Ishita Parikh, Stefan J. Green, Jared D. Hoffman, George Chlipala, M. Paul Murphy, Brent S. Sokola, Björn Bauer, Anika M. S. Hartz, and Ai-Ling Lin.

39. Pathophysiology of human visceral obesity: an update. NCBI *Physiol Rev. 2013* Jan;93(1):359-404. DOI: 10.1152/physrev.00033.2011. Tchernof A, Després JP.

40. Effect of weight loss and ketosis on postprandial cholecystokinin and free fatty acid concentrations. *Am J Clin Nutr.* 2008 May;87(5):1238-46. Chearskul S, Delbridge E, Shulkes A, Proietto J, Kriketos A.

41. Dietary influences on peripheral hormones regulating energy intake: potential applications for weight management. *J Am Diet Assoc.* 2005 Jul;105(7):1115-24. Orr J, Davy B.

42. Long-term dietary restriction influences plasma ghrelin and GOAT mRNA level in rats. *Physiol Behav.* 2010 Apr 19;99(5):605-

10. DOI: 10.1016/j.physbeh.2010.01.034. Epub 2010 Feb 9. Reimer RA, Maurer AD, Lau DC, Auer RN.

43. Gluconeogenesis and energy expenditure after a high-protein, carbohydrate-free diet. *Am J Clin Nutr.* 2009 Sep;90(3):519-26. DOI: 10.3945/ajcn.2009.27834. Epub 2009 Jul 29. Veldhorst MA, Westerterp- Plantenga MS, Westerterp KR.

44. Whey protein intake after resistance exercise activates mTOR signaling in a dose-dependent manner in human skeletal muscle. *Eur J Appl Physiol.* 2014 Apr;114(4):735-42. DOI: 10.1007/s00421-013- 2812-7. Epub 2014 Jan 3. Kakigi R, Yoshi-hara T, Ozaki H, Ogura Y, Ichinoseki-Sekine N, Kobayashi H, Naito H.

45. Effects of Dietary Composition on Energy Expenditure During Weight-Loss Maintenance *JAMA.* 2012;307(24):2627-2634. DOI:10.1001/jama.2012.6607. Cara B. Ebbeling, PhD; Janis F. Swain, MS, RD; Henry A. Feldman, PhD; et al William W. Wong, PhD; David L. Hachey, PhD; Erica Garcia-Lago, BA; David S. Lud-wig, MD, PhD

46. Effect of a high-fat Mediterranean diet on bodyweight and waist circumference: a prespecified secondary outcomes analysis of the PREDIMED randomized controlled trial. *Lancet Diabetes En-docrinol.* 2016 Aug;4(8):666-76. DOI: 10.1016/S2213-8587(16)30085-7. Epub 2016 Jun 6. Estruch R, Martínez-González MA, Corella D, Salas- Salvadó J, Fitó M, Chiva-Blanch G, Fiol M, Gómez-Gracia E, Arós F, Lapetra J, Serra-Majem L, Pintó X, Buil-Cosiales P, Sorlí JV, Muñoz MA, Basora-Gallisá J, Lamuela-Raventós RM, Serra-Mir M, Ros E, PREDIMED Study Investiga-tors.

47. A randomized trial comparing a very low carbohydrate diet and a calorie-restricted low fat diet on body weight and cardiovascu-lar risk factors in healthy women. *J Clin Endocrinol Metab.* 2003 Apr;88(4):1617-23. Brehm BJ, Seeley RJ, Daniels SR, D'Alessio DA.

48. Perceived hunger is lower and weight loss is greater in overweight premenopausal women consuming a low- carbohydrate/high-protein vs high-carbohydrate/low-fat diet. *J Am Diet Assoc.* 2005 Sep;105(9):1433-7. Nickols-Richardson SM, Coleman MD, Volpe JJ, Hosig KW.

Chapter 2

1. Longer fasts might help with weight loss but Americans eat all day long. *Los Angeles Times* Sep 24, 2015 | 11:55 AM By Melissa Healy

2. Calorie restriction is the most reasonable anti-ageing intervention: a meta-analysis of survival curves *Scientific Reports* Published: 10 April 2018 Yaru Liang, Chang Liu, Maoyang Lu, Qiongye Dong, Zimu Wang, Zhuoran Wang, Wenxiang Xiong, Nannan Zhang, Jiawei Zhou, Qingfei Liu, Xiaowo Wang & Zhao Wang

3. Effect of calorie restriction on energy expenditure in overweight and obese adult women. *Nutr Hosp.* 2015 Jun 1;31(6):2428-36. DOI: 10.3305/nh.2015.31.6.8782. Jiménez Jaime T, Leiva Balich L, Barrera Acevedo G, de la Maza Cave MP, Hirsch Birn S, Henríquez Parada S, Rodríguez Silva J, Bunout Barnett D.

4. Leptin, thyrotropin, and thyroid hormones in obese/overweight women before and after two levels of energy deficit. *Endocrine.* 2004 Jul;24(2):147-53. Kozłowska L, Rosołowska-Huszcz D.

5. Fasting enhances growth hormone secretion and amplifies the complex rhythms of growth hormone secretion in man. *J Clin Invest.* 1988 Apr; 81(4): 968–975. DOI: [10.1172/JCI113450] PMCID: PMC329619 PMID: 3127426 K Y Ho, J D Veldhuis, M L Johnson, R Furlanetto, W S Evans, K G Alberti, and M O Thorner.

6. Effect of intermittent fasting and refeeding on insulin action in healthy men. J Appl Physiol (1985). 2005 Dec;99(6):2128-36. Epub 2005 Jul 28. Halberg N, Henriksen M, Söderhamn N, Stallknecht B, Ploug T, Schjerling P, Dela F.

7. The effect of meal frequency in a reduced-energy regimen on the gastrointestinal and appetite hormones in patients with Type 2 diabetes: A randomized crossover study *PLoS One.* 2017; 12(4):

e0174820. Published online 2017 Apr 3. DOI: [10.1371/journal.pone.0174820] PMCID: PMC5378398 PMID: 28369078 Lenka Belinova, Hana Kahleova, Hana Malinska, Ondrej Topolcan, Jindra Windrichova, Olena Oliyarnyk, Ludmila Kazdova, Martin Hill, and Terezie Pelikanova, Dorit Samocha-Bonet, Editor

8. Meal frequency and timing in health and disease *Proc Natl Acad Sci U S A*. 2014 Nov 25; 111(47): 16647–16653. Published online 2014 Nov 17. DOI: [10.1073/pnas.1413965111] PMCID: PMC4250148 PMID: 25404320 Medical Sciences Mark P. Mattson, David B. Allison, Luigi Fontana, Michelle Harvie, Valter D. Longo, Willy J. Malaisse, Michael Mosley, Lucia Notterpek, Eric Ravussin, Frank A. J. L. Scheer, Thomas N. Seyfried, Krista A. Varady, and Satchidananda Panda.

9. Interleukin-6 contributes to early fasting-induced free fatty acid mobilization in mice. *Am J Physiol Regul Integr Comp Physiol*. 2014 Jun 1;306(11):R861-7. DOI: 10.1152/ajpregu.00533.2013. Epub 2014 Apr 2 Wueest S, Item F, Boyle CN, Jirkof P, Cesarovic N, Ellingsgaard H, Böni- Schnetzler M, Timper K, Arras M, Donath MY, Lutz TA, Schoenle EJ, Konrad D.

10. Fasting: molecular mechanisms and clinical applications. *Cell Metab*. 2014 Feb 4;19(2):181-92. DOI: 10.1016/j.cmet.2013.12.008. Epub 2014 Jan 16. Longo VD, Mattson MP.

11. Inverse relationship between brain glucose and ketone metabolism in adults during short-term moderate dietary ketosis: A dual tracer quantitative positron emission tomography study. *J Cereb Blood Flow Metab*. 2017 Jul;37(7):2485-2493. DOI: 10.1177/0271678X16669366. Epub 2016 Jan 1 Courchesne-Loyer A, Croteau E, Castellano CA, St-Pierre V, Hennebelle M, Cunnane SC.

12. Meal frequency and timing in health and disease *Proc Natl Acad Sci U S A*. 2014 Nov 25; 111(47): 16647–16653. Published online 2014 Nov 17. DOI: [10.1073/pnas.1413965111] PMCID: PMC4250148 PMID: 25404320 Medical Sciences Mark P. Mattson, David B. Allison, Luigi Fontana, Michelle Harvie, Valter

D. Longo, Willy J. Malaisse, Michael Mosley, Lucia Notterpek, Eric Ravussin, Frank A. J. L. Scheer, Thomas N. Seyfried, Krista A. Varady, and Satchidananda Panda.

13. Short-term fasting induces profound neuronal autophagy. 2010 Aug 16; 6(6): 702–710. Published online 2010 Aug 14. DOI: [10.4161/auto.6.6.12376] PMCID: PMC3106288 NIHMSID: NIHMS298250 PMID: 20534972 Mehrdad Alirezaei, Christopher C. Kemball, Claudia T. Flynn, Malcolm R. Wood, J. Lindsay Whitton, and William B. Kiosses.

14. Repetitive stimulation of autophagy-lysosome machinery by intermittent fasting preconditions the myocardium to ischemia-reperfusion injury *Autophagy*. 2015 Sep; 11(9): 1537–1560. Published online 2015 Jun 23. DOI: [10.1080/15548627.2015.1063768] PMCID: PMC4590628 PMID: 26103523 Rebecca J Godar, Xiucui Ma, Haiyan Liu, John T Murphy, Carla J Weinheimer, Attila Kovacs, Seth D Crosby, Paul Saftig, and Abhinav Diwan.

15. Impact of intermittent fasting on health and disease processes. *Ageing Res Rev. 2017* Oct;39:46-58. doi: 10.1016/j.arr.2016.10.005. Epub 2016 Oct 31. Mattson MP1, Longo VD2, Harvie M3.

16. Adipose, Bone Marrow and Synovial   Joint-Derived Mesenchymal Stem Cells for Cartilage Repair *Front Genet.* 2016; 7: 213. Published online 2016 Dec 20. DOI: [10.3389/fgene.2016.00213] PMCID: PMC5167763 PMID: 28066501 Christopher R. Fellows, Csaba Matta, Roza Zakany, Ilyas M. Khan, and Ali Mobasheri.

17. Nutrition and fasting mimicking diets in the prevention and treatment of autoimmune diseases and immunosenescence *Mol Cell Endocrinol.* 2017 Nov 5; 455: 4–12. Published online 2017 Jan 28. DOI: [10.1016/j.mce.2017.01.042] PMCID: PMC5862044 NIHMSID: NIHMS951053 PMID: 28137612 In Young Choi, Changhan Lee, and Valter D. Longo.

18. Prolonged fasting reduces IGF-1/PKA to promote hematopoietic-stem-cell-based regeneration and reverse immunosuppression. *Cell Stem Cell.* 2014 Jun 5;14(6):810-23. DOI:

10.1016/j.stem.2014.04.014. Cheng CW, Adams GB, Perin L, Wei M, Zhou X, Lam BS, Da Sacco S, Mirisola M, Quinn DI, Dorff TB, Kopchick JJ, Longo VD.

19. Diet mimicking fasting promotes regeneration and reduces auto-immunity and multiple sclerosis symptoms *Cell Rep.* 2016 Jun 7; 15(10): 2136–2146. Published online 2016 May 26. DOI: [10.1016/j.celrep.2016.05.009] PMCID: PMC4899145 NIHMSID: NIHMS785151 PMID: 27239035 In Young Choi, Laura Piccio, Patra Childress, Bryan Bollman, Arko Ghosh, Sebastian Brandhorst, Jorge Suarez, Andreas Michalsen, Anne H. Cross, Todd E. Morgan, Min Wei, Friedemann Paul, Markus Bock, and Valter D. Longo.

Chapter 3

1. Short-term fasting induces profound neuronal autophagy. 2010 Aug 16; 6(6): 702–710. Published online 2010 Aug 14. DOI: [10.4161/auto.6.6.12376] PMCID: PMC3106288 NIHMSID: NIHMS298250 PMID: 20534972 Mehrdad Alirezaei, Christopher C. Kemball, Claudia T. Flynn, Malcolm R. Wood, J. Lindsay Whitton, and William B. Kiosses.

2. Fasting: molecular mechanisms and clinical applications. *Cell Metab.* 2014 Feb 4;19(2):181-92. DOI: 10.1016/j.cmet.2013.12.008. Epub 2014 Jan 16 Longo VD, Mattson MP.

3. Metabolic Control of Autophagy *Cell.* 2014 Dec 4; 159(6): 1263–1276. DOI: [10.1016/j.cell.2014.11.006] PMCID: PMC4500936 NIHMSID: NIHMS704685 PMID: 25480292 Lorenzo Galluzzi, Federico Pietrocola, Beth Levine, and Guido Kroemer.

4. Preventing mutant huntingtin proteolysis and intermittent fasting promote autophagy in models of Huntington disease *Acta Neuropathol Commun.* 2018; 6: 16. Published online 2018 Mar 6. DOI: [10.1186/s40478-018-0518-0] PMCID: PMC5839066 PMID: 29510748 Dagmar E. Ehrnhoefer, Dale D. O. Martin, Mandi E. Schmidt, Xiaofan Qiu, Safia Ladha, Nicholas S. Caron, Niels H. Skotte, Yen T. N. Nguyen, Kuljeet Vaid, Amber L. Southwell, Sabine Engemann, Sonia Franciosi, and Michael R. Hayden.

5. Fasting enhances growth hormone secretion and amplifies the complex rhythms of growth hormone secretion in man. *J Clin Invest.* 1988 Apr; 81(4): 968–975. DOI: [10.1172/JCI113450] PMCID: PMC329619 PMID: 3127426 KY Ho, JD Veldhuis, ML Johnson, R Furlanetto, WS Evans, KG Alberti, and MO Thorner.

6. Effect of intermittent fasting and refeeding on insulin action in healthy men. *J Appl Physiol* (1985). 2005 Dec;99(6):2128-36. Epub 2005 Jul 28. Halberg N1, Henriksen M, Söderhamn N, Stallknecht B, Ploug T, Schjerling P, Dela F.

7. Calorie restriction is the most reasonable anti-aging intervention: a meta-analysis of survival curves *Scientific Reports* Published: 10 April 2018   Yaru Liang, Chang Liu, Maoyang Lu, Qiongye Dong, Zimu Wang, Zhuoran Wang, Wenxiang Xiong, Nannan Zhang, Jiawei Zhou, Qingfei Liu, Xiaowo Wang & Zhao Wang.

8. Anti-Aging Implications of Astragalus Membranaceus (Huangqi): A Well-Known Chinese Tonic *Aging Dis.* 2017 Dec; 8(6): 868–886. Published online 2017 Dec 1. DOI: [10.14336/AD.2017.0816] PMCID: PMC5758356 PMID: 29344421 Ping Liu, Haiping Zhao, and Yumin Luo.

9. The telomerase activator TA-65 elongates short telomeres and increases health span of adult/old mice without increasing cancer incidence. Aging Cell. 2011 Aug;10(4):604-21. DOI: 10.1111/j.1474-9726.2011.00700.x. Epub 2011 Apr 14. Bernardes de Jesus B, Schneeberger K, Vera E, Tejera A, Harley CB, Blasco MA.

10. Calorie restriction extends yeast life span by lowering the level of NADH. *Genes Dev.* 2004 Jan 1;18(1):12-6. Lin SJ, Ford E, Haigis M, Liszt G, Guarente L.

11. Fasting activates macroautophagy in neurons of Alzheimer's disease mouse model but is insufficient to degrade amyloid-beta. *Sci Rep.* 2015 Jul 14;5:12115. DOI: 10.1038/srep12115. Chen X, Kondo K, Motoki K, Homma H, Okazawa H.

12. Oxaloacetate supplementation increases lifespan in Caenorhabditis elegans through an AMPK/FOXO-dependent pathway. *Aging*

Cell. 2009 Dec;8(6):765-8. DOI: 10.1111/j.1474-9726.2009.00527.x. Epub 2009 Sep 30. Williams DS, Cash A, Hamadani L, Diemer T.

13. Oxaloacetate Enhances Neuronal Cell Bioenergetic Fluxes and Infrastructure *J Neurochem.* 2016 Apr; 137(1): 76–87. Published online 2016 Mar 11. DOI: [10.1111/jnc.13545] PMCID: PMC5482267 NIHMSID: NIHMS865868 PMID: 26811028 Heather M. Wilkins, Scott Koppel, Steven M. Carl, Suruchi Ramanujan, Ian Weidling, Mary L. Michaelis, Elias K. Michaelis, and Russell H. Swerdlow.

14. Oxaloacetic Acid Supplementation as a Mimic of Calorie Restriction *Open Longevity Science*, 2009, 3: 22-27 Alan Cash Terra Biological LLC, 5033 Seachase Street, San Diego, CA 92130, USA Electronic publication date 03/11/2009 [DOI: 10.2174/1876326X00903010022]

15. Alternate-day versus daily energy restriction diets: which is more effective for weight loss? A systematic review and meta-analysis. *Obes Sci Pract.* 2016 Sep;2(3):293-302. Epub 2016 Jul 15. Alhamdan BA, Garcia-Alvarez A, Alzahrnai AH, Karanxha J, Stretchberry DR, Contrera KJ, Utria AF, Cheskin LJ.

16. Longer daily fasting times improve health and longevity in mice. *National Institute on Aging*, September 2018, https://www.nia.nih.gov/news/longer-daily-fasting-times-improve-health- and-longevity-mice, Chip Rose.

17. Daily Fasting Improves Health and Survival in Male Mice Independent of Diet Composition and Calories. *Cell Metab. 2018* Aug 24. pii: S1550-4131(18)30512-6. DOI: 10.1016/j.cmet.2018.08.011. Mitchell SJ, Bernier M, Mattison JA, Aon MA, Kaiser TA, Anson RM, Ikeno Y, Anderson RM, Ingram DK, de Cabo R.

18. What's the Deal with 'Toxins' in Coffee? *Dr. Dan Pompa YouTube Episode 182* November 17, 2017 // by Dr. Daniel Pompa, PSc.D//

Chapter 4

1. Diet, individual responsiveness and cancer prevention. *The Journal of Nutrition.* 2003 Jul;133(7):2400S-2403S. DOI: 10.1093/jn/133.7.2400S. Wargovich MJ, Cunningham JE.

2. Scientific American. July, 2018. https://www.scientificamerican.com/magazine/sa/2018/07-01/.

3. Fasting enhances growth hormone secretion and amplifies the complex rhythms of growth hormone secretion in man. *J Clin Invest.* 1988 Apr; 81(4): 968–975. DOI: [10.1172/JCI113450] PMCID: PMC329619 PMID: 3127426 KY Ho, JD Veldhuis, ML Johnson, R Furlanetto, WS Evans, KG Alberti, and MO Thorner.

4. Effect of intermittent fasting and refeeding on insulin action in healthy men. *J Appl Physiol* (1985). 2005 Dec;99(6):2128-36. Epub 2005 Jul 28 Halberg N, Henriksen M, Söderhamn N, Stallknecht B, Ploug T, Schjerling P, Dela F.

5. Anti-inflammatory effects of noradrenaline on LPS-treated microglial cells: Suppression of NFκB nuclear translocation and subsequent STAT1 phosphorylation. *Neurochem Int.* 2015 Nov;90:56- 66. DOI: 10.1016/j.neuint.2015.07.010. Epub 2015 Jul 16. Ishii Y, Yamaizumi A, Kawakami A, Islam A, Choudhury ME, Takahashi H, Yano H, Tanaka J.

6. Anti-inflammatory effects of noradrenaline on LPS-treated microglial cells: Suppression of NFκB nuclear translocation and subsequent STAT1 phosphorylation. *Neurochem Int.* 2015 Nov;90:56- 66. DOI: 10.1016/j.neuint.2015.07.010. Epub 2015 Jul 16. Ishii Y, Yamaizumi A, Kawakami A, Islam A, Choudhury ME, Takahashi H, Yano H, Tanaka J.

7. The effect of norepinephrine on the energetic metabolism of heart muscle. *Exp Med Surg.* 1968;26(1-2):15-20. Bachledová E, Gvozdják J, Niederland TR, Hocman G.

8. Modulation of amino acid neurotransmitter actions by other neurotransmitters *Canadian Journal of Physiology and Pharma-*

cology, 1991, 69(7): 1115-1122, https://doi.org/10.1139/y91-163 Kenneth C. Marshall and Huangui Xiong

9. Mood is indirectly related to serotonin, norepinephrine and dopamine levels in humans: a meta-analysis of monoamine depletion studies. *Mol Psychiatry*. 2007 Apr;12(4):331-59. Epub 2007 Jan 16.

10. Ibid.

11. The action of norepinephrine in the rat hippocampus. I. Iontophoretic studies *Science Direct*, Volume 72, Issue 1, 31 May 1974, Pages 79-97 Author links open overlay panel Menahem Segal, Floyd E.Bloom.

12. Gut Microbiota Orchestrates Energy Homeostasis during Cold. *Cell*. 2015 Dec 3;163(6):1360-74. doi: 10.1016/j.cell.2015.11.004. Chevalier C, Stojanović O, Suarez-Zamorano N, Tarallo V, Veyrat-Durebex C, Rigo D, Fabbiano S, Stevanović A.

13. Fasting enhances growth hormone secretion and amplifies the complex rhythms of growth hormone secretion in man. *J Clin Invest*. 1988 Apr;81(4):968-75. Ho KY, Veldhuis JD, Johnson ML, Furlanetto R, Evans WS, Alberti KG, Thorner MO.

14. Effects of weight loss via high fat vs. low fat alternate day fasting diets on free fatty acid profiles. *Sci Reports*. 2015 Jan 5;5:7561. DOI: 10.1038/srep07561. Varady KA, Dam VT, Klempel MC, Horne M, Cruz R, Kroeger CM, Santosa S.

15. The effects of intermittent or continuous energy restriction on weight loss and metabolic disease risk markers: a randomized trial in young overweight women. *Int J Obes* (Lond). 2011 May;35(5):714-27. DOI: 10.1038/ijo.2010.171. Epub 2010 Oct 5. Harvie MN, Pegington M, Mattson MP, Frystyk J, Dillon B, Evans G, Cuzick J, Jebb SA, Martin B, Cutler RG, Son TG, Maudsley S, Carlson OD, Egan JM, Flyvbjerg A, Howell A. axis in obese men during short-term fasting. *Acta Endocrinol* (Copenh). 1989 Nov;121(5):727-32. Röjdmark S, Asplund A, Rössner S.

16. The effect of dietary composition and of insulin on gluconeogenesis in rainbow trout (Salmo gairdneri) *The British Journal of Nutrition* November 1977, pp. 385-395 https://doi.org/ 10.1079/BJN19770103 Published online: 09 March 2007. CB Cowey, M. De La Higuera, and J. W. Adron.

17. Effect of intermittent fasting and refeeding on insulin action in healthy men *Journal of Applied PhysiologyVol. 99, No.* 6 01 Dec 2005https://doi.org/10.1152/japplphysiol.00683.2005

18. Nils Halberg, Morten Henriksen, Nathalie Söderhamn, Bente Stallknecht, Thorkil Ploug, Peter Schjerling, and Flemming Dela.

19. Insulin and insulin signaling play a critical role in fat induction of insulin resistance in mouse *Am J Physiol Endocrinol Metab.* 2011 Aug; 301(2): E391–E401. Published online 2011 May 17. DOI: [10.1152/ajpendo.00164.2011] PMCID: PMC3154527 PMID: 21586696 Jie Ning, Tao Hong, Xuefeng Yang, Shuang Mei, Zhenqi Liu, Hui-Yu Liu, and Wenhong Cao.

20. Leucine-enriched essential amino acid and carbohydrate ingestion following resistance exercise enhances mTOR signaling and protein synthesis in human muscle *American Journal of Physiology-Endocrinology and MetabolismVol. 294, No. 2* 01 Feb 2008https://doi.org/10.1152/ajpendo.00582.2007 Hans C. Dreyer, Micah J. Drummond, Bart Pennings, Satoshi Fujita, Erin L. Glynn, David L. Chinkes, Shaheen Dhanani, Elena Volpi, and Blake B. Rasmussen.

21. mTOR signaling at a glance *Journal of Cell Science* 2009 122: 3589-3594; DOI: 10.1242/jcs.051011 Mathieu Laplante, David M. Sabatini.

22. Interventions to Slow Aging in Humans: Are We Ready? *Aging Cell.* 2015 Aug;14(4):497-510. DOI: 10.1111/acel.12338. Epub 2015 Apr Longo VD, Antebi A, Bartke A, Barzilai N, Brown-Borg HM, Caruso C, Curiel TJ, de Cabo R, Franceschi C, Gems D, Ingram DK, Johnson TE, Kennedy BK, Kenyon C, Klein S, Kopchick JJ, Lepperdinger G, Madeo F, Mirisola MG, Mitchell JR, Passarino G,

Rudolph KL, Sedivy JM, Shadel GS, Sinclair DA, Spindler SR, Suh Y, Vijg J, Vinciguerra M, Fontana L.

23. Autophagy: renovation of cells and tissues *Cell. 2011* Nov 11; 147(4):728-41. DOI: 10.1016/j.cell.2011.10.026. Mizushima N, Komatsu M.

24. Insulin: understanding its action in health and disease. Br J Anaesth. 2000 Jul;85(1):69-79. Sonksen P, Sonksen J.

25. The effect of dietary composition and of insulin on gluconeogenesis in rainbow trout (Salmo gairdneri) *Volume 38, Issue 3* Nov 1977, pp. 385-395 https://doi.org/10.1079/BJN19770103 Published online: 09 March 2007 CB Cowey, M. De La Higuera, and JW Adron. Institute of Marine Biochemistry, St Fitticks Road, Aberdeen AB1 3RA

26. Gluconeogenesis and energy expenditure after a high-protein, carbohydrate-free diet. *Am J Clin Nutr.* 2009 Sep;90(3):519-26. DOI: 10.3945/ajcn.2009.27834. Epub 2009 Jul 29. Veldhorst MA1, Westerterp- Plantenga MS, Westerterp KR. Ann. N.Y. Acad. Sci. ISSN 0077-8923

27. Insulin regulation of gluconeogenesis *ANNALS OF THE NEW YORK ACADEMY OF SCIENCES* Issue: The Year in Diabetes and Obesity REVIEW Maximilian Hatting, Clint D.J. Tavares, Kfir Sharabi, Amy K. Rines, and Pere Puigserver

    a. Department of Cancer Biology, Dana-Farber Cancer Institute, Boston, Massachusetts.

    b. Department of Cell Biology, Harvard Medical School, Boston, Massachusetts, Address for correspondence: Dr. Pere Puigserver, Department of Cancer Biology, Dana-Farber Cancer Institute, 450 Brookline Av., CLSB-11144, Boston, MA 02215. pere_puigserver@dfci.harvard.edu

28. Effect of physiological hyperinsulinemia on gluconeogenesis in nondiabetic subjects and in Type 2 diabetic patients. *Diabetes. 2001* Aug;50(8):1807-12. Gastaldelli A, Toschi E, Pettiti M, Frascerra S, Quiñones-Galvan A, Sironi AM, Natali A, Ferrannini E.

29. Insulin: understanding its action in health and disease *BJA: British Journal of Anaesthesia*, Volume 85, Issue 1, 1 July 2000, Pages 69–79, https://doi.org/10.1093/bja/85.1.69 Published: 01 July 2000. P Sonksen, J Sonksen.

30. Insulin regulation of gluconeogenesis. *Ann N Y Acad Sci.* 2018 Jan;1411(1):21-35. DOI: 10.1111/nyas.13435. Epub 2017 Sep 3. Hatting M, Tavares CDJ, Sharabi K, Rines AK, Puigserver P.

31. Nutritional Ketosis and Mitohormesis: Potential Implications for Mitochondrial Function and Human Health *J Nutr Metab.* 2018; 2018: 5157645. Published online 2018 Feb 11. DOI: [10.1155/2018/ 5157645] PMCID: PMC5828461 PMID: 29607218 Vincent J. Miller, Frederick A. Villamena, and Jeff S. Volek .

32. Prolonged fasting reduces IGF-1/PKA to promote hematopoietic-stem-cell-based regeneration and reverse immunosuppression. *Cell Stem Cell.* 2014 Jun 5;14(6):810-23.

    DOI: 10.1016/j.stem.2014.04.014. Cheng CW, Adams GB, Perin L, Wei M, Zhou X, Lam BS, Da Sacco S, Mirisola M, Quinn DI, Dorff TB, Kopchick JJ, Longo VD.

33. Intermittent Fasting – The Best Strategy for Weight Loss Articles » *Intermittent Fasting – The Best Strategy for Weight Loss* February 13, 2018 // by Dr. Daniel Pompa, PSc.D

34. Fasting for three days can regenerate entire immune system, study finds *The Telegraph News/Science* 5 June 2014 • 7:45pm by Sarah Knapton, Science Correspondent

Chapter 5

1. Diet, individual responsiveness and cancer prevention *J Nutr.* 2003 Jul;133(7 Suppl):2400S-2403S. DOI: 10.1093/jn/133.7.2400S. Wargovich MJ1, Cunningham JE.

2. Nutritional Ketosis and Mitohormesis: Potential Implications for Mitochondrial Function and Human Health *J Nutr Metab. 2018*; 2018: 5157645. Published online 2018 Feb 11. DOI: [10.1155/2018/ 5157645] PMCID: PMC5828461 PMID:

29607218 Vincent J. Miller, Frederick A. Villamena, and Jeff S. Volek

Chapter 6

1. Autophagy in stem cells *Autophagy.* 2013 Jun 1; 9(6): 830–849. Published online 2013 Mar 13. DOI: [10.4161/auto.24132] PMCID: PMC3672294 PMID: 23486312 Jun-Lin Guan, Anna Katharina Simon, Mark Prescott, Javier A. Menendez, Fei Liu, Fen Wang, Chenran Wang, Ernst Wolvetang, Alejandro Vazquez-Martin, and Jue Zhang.

2. Prolonged fasting reduces IGF-1/PKA to promote hematopoietic-stem-cell-based regeneration and reverse immunosuppression. *Cell Stem Cell.* 2014 Jun 5;14(6):810-23. DOI: 10.1016/j.stem.2014.04.014. Cheng CW, Adams GB, Perin L, Wei M, Zhou X, Lam BS, Da Sacco S, Mirisola M, Quinn DI, Dorff TB, Kopchick JJ, Longo VD.

3. Fasting enhances growth hormone secretion and amplifies the complex rhythms of growth hormone secretion in man. *J Clin Invest.* 1988 Apr; 81(4): 968–975. DOI: [10.1172/JCI113450] PMCID: PMC329619 PMID: 3127426 KY Ho, JD Veldhuis, ML Johnson, R Furlanetto, WS Evans, KG Alberti, and MO Thorner.

4. Autophagy: Renovation of Cells and Tissues *Science Direct,* Cell,Volume 147, Issue 4, 11 November 2011, Pages 728-741. Author Noboru Mizushima, Masaaki Komatsu

5. Fasting-Mimicking Diet Promotes Ngn3-Driven β-Cell Regeneration to Reverse Diabetes. *Cell.* 2017 Feb 23;168(5):775- 788.e12. DOI: 10.1016/j.cell.2017.01.040. Cheng CW, Villani V, Buono R, Wei M, Kumar S, Yilmaz OH, Cohen P, Sneddon JB, Perin L, Longo VD.

6. Ibid.

7. Stem Cells *Medicine Net,* https://www.medicinenet.com/stem_cells/ article.htm. Medical Author: Melissa Conrad Stöppler, MD Medical Editor: William C. Shiel Jr., MD, FACP, FACR.

8. Fasting Activates Fatty Acid Oxidation to Enhance Intestinal Stem Cell Function during Homeostasis and Aging. *Cell Stem Cell.* 2018 May 3;22(5):769-778.e4. DOI: 10.1016/j.stem.2018.04.001. Mihaylova MM, Cheng CW, Cao AQ, Tripathi S, Mana MD, Bauer-Rowe KE, Abu-Remaileh M, Clavain L, Erdemir A, Lewis CA, Freinkman E, Dickey AS, La Spada AR, Huang Y, Bell GW, Deshpande V, Carmeliet P, Katajisto P, Sabatini DM, Yilmaz ÖH.

9. Prolonged fasting reduces IGF-1/PKA to promote hematopoietic-stem-cell-based regeneration and reverse immunosuppression. *Cell Stem Cell.* 2014 Jun 5;14(6):810-23. DOI: 10.1016/j.stem.2014.04.014. Cheng CW, Adams GB, Perin L, Wei M, Zhou X, Lam BS, Da Sacco S, Mirisola M, Quinn DI, Dorff TB, Kopchick JJ, Longo VD.

10. The biochemistry of natural fasting at its limits. *Experientia.* 1992 Jun 15;48(6):575-82. Castellini M, Rea LD.

11. Ibid.

12. Effect of intermittent fasting and refeeding on insulin action in healthy men. *J Appl Physiol* (1985). 2005 Dec;99(6):2128-36. Epub 2005 Jul 28. Halberg N1, Henriksen M, Söderhamn N, Stallknecht B, Ploug T, Schjerling P, Dela F.

13. Ibid.

14. Increased gut microbiota diversity and abundance of Faecalibacterium prausnitzii and Akkermansia after fasting: a pilot study *Wien Klin Wochenschr.* 2015; 127(9-10): 394–398. Published online 2015 Mar 13. DOI: [10.1007/s00508-015-0755-1] PMCID: PMC4452615 PMID: 25763563 Marlene Remely, Berit Hippe, Isabella Geretschlaeger, Sonja Stegmayer, Ingrid Hoefinger, and Alexander Haslberger

15. Effect of caloric restriction on gut permeability, inflammation markers, and fecal microbiota in obese women Article (PDF Available) in *Scientific Reports* 7(1). December 2017 DOI: 10.1038/ s41598-017-12109-9 Beate Brandl, Technische Universität München, Thomas Skurk, Technische Universität Mün-

chen, Ljiljana Hastreiter Ilias Lagkouvardos, Technische Universität München, Sandra Fischer, Technische Universität München, Janine Büttner,Charité Universitätsmedizin Berlin, Teresa Kellerer, Universität München, Thomas Clavel, RWTH University Hospital, Michael Rychlik, Technische Universität München, Dirk Haller, Technische Universität München, Hans Hauner.

16. Neuronal energy-sensing pathway promotes energy balance by modulating disease tolerance *Proceedings of The National Academy of Sciences* PNAS June 7, 2016 113 (23) E3307-E3314; published ahead of print May 20, 2016 https://doi.org/10.1073/pnas.1606106113 Run Shen, Biao Wang, Maria G. Giribaldi, Janelle Ayres, John B. Thomas, and Marc Montminy. Contributed by Marc Montminy, April 18, 2016 (sent for review March 1, 2016; reviewed by Ethan Bier and Jongkyeong Chung)

17. Effects of fasting and refeeding on ob gene expression in white adipose tissue of lean and obese (ob/ob) mice *Science Direct* FEBS Letters Volume 368, Issue 3, 24 July 1995, Pages 488-490 Paul Trayhurn, Moira EA Thomas, Jacqueline S Duncan, D Vernon Rayner.

18. Epigenetics: the language of the cell? *Epigenomics.* 2014 Feb;6(1):73-88. DOI: 10.2217/epi.13.72. Huang B1, Jiang C, Zhang R.

19. Ibid.

20. Ibid.

21. Ibid.

22. Ibid.

23. Nutrition and fasting mimicking diets in the prevention and treatment of autoimmune diseases and immunosenescence. *Mol Cell Endocrinol.* 2017 Nov 5;455:4-12. DOI: 10.1016/j.mce.2017.01.042. Epub 2017 Jan 28. Choi IY, Lee C, Longo VD.

24. The ketogenic diet reverses gene expression patterns and reduces reactive oxygen species levels when used as an adjuvant therapy for glioma. *Nutr Metab (Lond).* 2010 Sep 10;7:74. doi: 10.1186/1743-7075-7-74. Stafford P1, Abdelwahab MG, Kim DY, Preul MC, Rho JM, Scheck AC.

25. Fasting: molecular mechanisms and clinical applications. *Cell Metab.* 2014 Feb 4;19(2):181-92. DOI: 10.1016/j.cmet.2013.12.008. Epub 2014 Jan 16. Longo VD, Mattson MP.

26. Body weight loss increases plasma and adipose tissue concentrations of potentially toxic pollutants in obese individuals. *The International Journal of Obesity* Published: 27 September 2000 International Journal of Obesity volume 24, pages 1272–1278 (2000) Chevrier, É Dewailly, P Ayotte, P Mauriège, J-P Després & A Tremblay.

27. Autophagy: renovation of cells and tissues. *Cell.* 2011 Nov 11;147(4):728-41. DOI: 10.1016/j.cell.2011.10.026. Mizushima N, Komatsu M.

28. Prolonged fasting reduces IGF-1/PKA to promote hematopoietic-stem-cell-based regeneration and reverse immunosuppression. *Cell Stem Cell.* 2014 Jun 5;14(6):810-23. DOI: 10.1016/j.stem.2014.04.014. Cheng CW, Adams GB, Perin L, Wei M, Zhou X, Lam BS, Da Sacco S, Mirisola M, Quinn DI, Dorff TB, Kopchick JJ, Longo VD.

29. Fasting enhances growth hormone secretion and amplifies the complex rhythms of growth hormone secretion in man. *The Journal of Clinical Investigation* First published April 1, 1988 Free access | 10.1172/JCI113450 https://www.jci.org/articles/view/113450. KY Ho, JD Veldhuis, ML Johnson, R Furlanetto, WS Evans, KG Alberti, and MO Thorner.

30. Protein and amino acid restriction, aging and disease: from yeast to humans. *Trends Endocrinol Metab.* 2014 Nov;25(11):558-66.

DOI: 10.1016/j.tem.2014.07.002. Epub 2014 Aug 19. Mirzaei H, Suarez JA, Longo VD.

31. A Diet Mimicking Fasting Promotes Regeneration and Reduces Autoimmunity and Multiple Sclerosis Symptoms. *Cell Rep.* 2016 Jun 7;15(10):2136-2146. DOI: 10.1016/j.celrep.2016.05.009. Epub 2016 May Choi IY, Piccio L, Childress P, Bollman B, Ghosh A, Brandhorst S, Suarez J, Michalsen A, Cross AH, Morgan TE, Wei M, Paul F, Bock M6, Longo VD.

32. Fasting-mimicking diet and markers/risk factors for aging, diabetes, cancer, and cardiovascular disease. *Sci Transl Med.* 2017 Feb 15;9(377). pii: eaai8700. DOI: 10.1126/scitranslmed.aai8700. Wei M, Brandhorst S, Shelehchi M, Mirzaei H, Cheng CW, Budniak J, Groshen S, Mack WJ, Guen E, Di Biase S, Cohen P, Morgan TE, Dorff T, Hong K, Michalsen A, Laviano A, Longo VD.

33. Ibid.

34. PROLON-Benefits of a Fasting Mimicking Diet website link for *PROLON* https://prolonfmd.com/af/?affID=1023&offerID=3

35. **Fasting-Mimicking** ieDt   Promotesgn3-NDriven β-Cell Regeneration to Reverse Diabetes *Science Direct,* Cell Volume 168, Issue 5, 23 ebFruary 2017, Pages 775-788. Volume 168, ssIue 5, 23February 2017, Pages 75-788.e12 Chia-WeiCheng, ValentinaVillani, Roberta Buono, MinWei, SanjeevKumar, Omer H.Yilmaz, PinchasCohen, Julie B.Sneddon, LauraPerin, Valter D.Longo.

36. Cancer as a metabolic disease: implications for novel therapeutics. *Carcinogenesis.* 2014 Mar;35(3):515-27. DOI: 10.1093/ carcin/bgt480. Epub 2013 Dec 16. Seyfried TN1, Flores RE, Poff AM, D'Agostino DP.

37. Metabolic therapy: a new paradigm for managing malignant brain cancer. *Cancer Lett.* 2015 Jan 28;356(2 Pt A):289-300. DOI: 10.1016/j.canlet.2014.07.015. Epub 2014 Jul 25. Seyfried TN, Flores R, Poff AM, D'Agostino DP, Mukherjee P.

38. A fasting inducible switch modulates gluconeogenesis via activator/coactivator exchange *Nature, International Journal of Science*, volume 456, pages 269–273 (13 November 2008) Published: 05 October 2008 Yi Liu, Renaud Dentin, Danica Chen, Susan Hedrick, Kim Ravnskjaer, Simon Schenk, Jill Milne, David J. Meyers, Phil Cole, John Yates III, Jerrold Olefsky, Leonard Guarente & Marc Montminy

39. Gluconeogenesis and hepatic glycogenolysis during exercise at the lactate threshold. *J Appl Physiol* (1985). 2013 Feb;114(3):297-306. DOI: 10.1152/japplphysiol.01202.2012. Epub 2012 Dec 13. Emhoff CA, Messonnier LA, Horning MA, Fattor JA, Carlson TJ, Brooks GA.

40. Cortisol-Induced Insulin Resistance in Man: Impaired Suppression of Glucose Production and Stimulation of Glucose Utilization due to a Postreceptor Defect of Insulin Action* *The Journal of Clinical Endocrinology & Metabolism*, Volume 54, Issue 1, 1 January 1982, Pages 131–138, https://doi.org/10.1210/jcem-54-1-131. Robert A. Rizza, Lawrence J. Mandarino, John E. Gerich Author Notes.

41. Fasting enhances growth hormone secretion and amplifies the complex rhythms of growth hormone secretion in man. *J Clin Invest.* 1988 Apr;81(4):968-75. Ho KY, Veldhuis JD, Johnson ML, Furlanetto R, Evans WS, Alberti KG, Thorner MO.

42. Short-term fasting induces profound neuronal autophagy. 2010 Aug 16; 6(6): 702–710. Published online 2010 Aug 14. DOI: [10.4161/auto.6.6.12376] PMCID: PMC3106288 NIHMSID: NIHMS298250 PMID: 20534972 Mehrdad Alirezaei, Christopher C. Kemball, Claudia T. Flynn, Malcolm R. Wood, J. Lindsay Whitton, and William B. Kiosses.

43. Fasting: molecular mechanisms and clinical applications. *Cell Metab.* 2014 Feb 4;19(2):181-92. DOI: 10.1016/j.cmet.2013.12.008. Epub 2014 Jan 16. Longo VD, Mattson MP

44. Ibid.

45. Prolonged fasting reduces IGF-1/PKA to promote hematopoietic-stem-cell-based regeneration and reverse immunosuppression. *Cell Stem Cell.* 2014 Jun 5;14(6):810-23. DOI: 10.1016/j.stem.2014.04.014. Cheng CW, Adams GB, Perin L, Wei M, Zhou X, Lam BS, Da Sacco S, Mirisola M, Quinn DI, Dorff TB, Kopchick JJ, Longo VD.

46. Effects of fasting and refeeding on ob gene expression in white adipose tissue of lean and obese (ob/ob) mice. *Science Direct* FEBS Letters Volume 368, Issue 3, 24 July 1995, Pages 488-490. PaulTrayhurn, Moira EA, Thomas Jacqueline, S Duncan, D Vernon Rayner. https://doi.org/10.1016/0014-5793(95)00719-P.

47. Ketogenic diet enhances neurovascular function with altered gut microbiome in young healthy mice. *Sci Rep.* 2018; 8: 6670. Published online 2018 Apr 27. DOI: [10.1038/s41598-018-25190-5] PMCID: PMC5923270 PMID: 29703936 David Ma,1 Amy C. Wang,1 Ishita Parikh,1 Stefan J. Green,2 Jared D. Hoffman,1,3 George Chlipala,2 M. Paul Murphy,1,4 Brent S. Sokola,5 Björn Bauer, Anika MS Hartz, and Ai- Ling Lin.

48. Ibid.

49. Dietary ketosis enhances memory in mild cognitive impairment. *Neurobiol Aging.* Author manuscript; available in PMC 2013 Feb 1. Published in final edited form as: Neurobiol Aging. 2012 Feb; 33(2): 425.e19–425.e27. Published online 2010 Dec 3. DOI: [10.1016/j.neurobiolaging.2010.10.006] PMCID: PMC3116949 NIHMSID: NIHMS246883 PMID: 21130529 Robert Krikorian, Marcelle D Shidler, Krista Dangelo, Sarah C Couch, Stephen C Benoit, and Deborah J Clegg.

50. Ketogenic diet for treatment of intractable epilepsy in adults: A meta-analysis of observational studies. *Epilepsia Open.* 2018 Feb 19;3(1):9-17. DOI: 10.1002/epi4.12098. eCollection 2018 Mar. Liu H, Yang Y, Wang Y, Tang H, Zhang F, Zhang Y, Zhao Y.

51. Glucose Levels and Risk of Dementia. *The New England Journal of Medicine* August 8, 2013 N Engl J Med 2013; 369:540-548 DOI: 10.1056/NEJMoa1215740 Paul K Crane, MD, MPH, Rod Walker,

MS, Rebecca A. Hubbard, PhD, Ge Li, MD, PhD, David M. Nathan, MD, Hui Zheng, PhD, Sebastien Haneuse, PhD, Suzanne Craft, PhD, Thomas J. Montine, MD, PhD, Steven E. Kahn, MB, ChB, Wayne McCormick, MD, MPH, Susan M. McCurry, PhD, James D. Bowen, MD, and Eric B. Larson, MD, MPH.

52. Ibid.

53. Low-fat versus ketogenic diet in Parkinson's disease: A pilot randomized controlled trial. *The Official Journal of the International Parkinson and Movement Disorder Society* FRACP First published: 11 August 2018 https://doi.org/10.1002/mds.27390 Matthew CL Phillips MSc, FRACP, Deborah KJ Murtagh, Linda J Gilbertson BLitComm, PGCert(Nursing), Fredrik J.S. Asztely PhD.

54. Crohn's disease successfully treated with the paleolithic ketogenic diet. *ResearchGate https://www.researchgate.net/publication/ 306373055_Crohn's_disease_suc cessful- ly_treated_with_the_paleolithic_ketogenic_diet* Article (PDF Available). September 2016 with 18,577 Reads DOI: 10.5348/ijcri-2016102- CR-10690 Csaba Tót -International Center for Medical Nutritional Intervention, Andrea Dabóczi-Paleomedicina Hungary, Mark Howard, Nicholas J. Miller, Zsofia Clemens-Paleomedicina Hungary.

55. Fasting enhances growth hormone secretion and amplifies the complex rhythms of growth hormone secretion in man. *J Clin Invest.* 1988 Apr;81(4):968-75. Ho KY1, Veldhuis JD, Johnson ML, Furlanetto R, Evans WS, Alberti KG, Thorner MO.

56. The effect of intermittent energy and carbohydrate restriction v. daily energy restriction on weight loss and metabolic disease risk markers in overweight women. *Br J Nutr.* 2013 Oct;110(8):1534-47. DOI: 10.1017/S0007114513000792. Epub 2013 Apr 16. Harvie M, Wright C, Pegington M, McMullan D, Mitchell E, Martin B, Cutler RG, Evans G, Whiteside S, Maudsley S, Camandola S, Wang R, Carlson OD, Egan JM, Mattson MP, Howell A.

57. Diet mimicking fasting promotes regeneration and reduces auto-immunity and multiple sclerosis symptoms. *Cell Rep.* 2016 Jun 7; 15(10): 2136–2146.Published online 2016 May 26. DOI: [10.1016/ j.celrep.2016.05.009] PMCID: PMC4899145 NIHMSID: NIHMS785151 PMID: 27239035 In Young Choi, Laura Piccio, Patra Childress, Bryan Bollman, Arko Ghosh, Sebastian Brandhorst, Jorge Suarez, Andreas Michalsen, Anne H. Cross, Todd E. Morgan, Min Wei, Friedemann Paul, Markus Bock, and Valter D. Longo.

58. The effect of intermittent energy and carbohydrate restriction v. daily energy restriction on weight loss and metabolic disease risk markers in overweight women. *Br J Nutr.* 2013 Oct;110(8):1534-47. DOI: 10.1017/S0007114513000792. Epub 2013 Apr 16. Harvie M1, Wright C, Pegington M, McMullan D, Mitchell E, Martin B, Cutler RG, Evans G, Whiteside S, Maudsley S, Camandola S, Wang R, Carlson OD, Egan JM, Mattson MP, Howell A.

59. Prolonged fasting reduces IGF-1/PKA to promote hematopoietic-stem-cell-based regeneration and reverse immunosuppression. *Cell Stem Cell.* 2014 Jun 5;14(6):810-23. DOI: 10.1016/j.stem.2014.04.014. Cheng CW, Adams GB, Perin L, Wei M, Zhou X, Lam BS, Da Sacco S, Mirisola M, Quinn DI, Dorff TB, Kopchick JJ, Longo VD.

60. A general introduction to the biochemistry of mitochondrial fatty acid β-oxidation *Journal of Inherited Metabolic Disease* October 2010, Volume 33, Issue 5, pp 469–477. Authors and affiliations Sander Michel Houten, Ronald J. A. Wanders. Nutritional Ketosis and Mitohormesis: Potential Implications for Mitochondrial Function and Human Health. *J Nutr Metab.* 2018; 2018: 5157645. Published online 2018 Feb 11. DOI: [10.1155/2018/ 5157645] PMCID: PMC5828461 PMID: 29607218

61. Vincent J. Miller, Frederick A. Villamena, and Jeff S. Volek, corresponding author.

62. Body weight loss increases plasma and adipose tissue concentrations of potentially toxic pollutants in obese individuals. *International Journal of Obesity* volume 24, pages 1272–1278 (2000)

Published: 27 September 2000 J Chevrier, É Dewailly, P Ayotte, P Mauriège, J-P Després & A Tremblay.

63. Autophagy: renovation of cells and tissues. *Cell.* 2011 Nov 11;147(4):728-41. DOI: 10.1016/j.cell.2011.10.026. Mizushima N1, Komatsu M.

64. Thyroidal dysfunction and environmental chemicals—potential impact on brain development. *Environ Health Perspect.* 2000 Jun; 108(Suppl 3): 433–438. DOI: [10.1289/ehp.00108s3433] PMCID: PMC1637839 PMID: 10852841 Research Article. S P Porterfield.

65. Determination of Mitochondrial Membrane Potential and Reactive Oxygen Species in Live Rat Cortical Neurons. *J Vis Exp.* 2011; (51): 2704. Published online 2011 May 23. DOI: [10.3791/2704] PMCID: PMC3143685 PMID: 21654619. Dinesh C. Joshi, and Joanna C. Bakowska.

66. Role of fat-derived substrates in the regulation of gluconeogenesis during fasting. *The American Journal of Physiology* F. Fery, L. Plat, C. Melot, and EO Balasse. 01 May 1996https://doi.org/10.1152/ajpendo.1996.270.5.E822

67. Fasting: molecular mechanisms and clinical applications. *Cell Metab.* 2014 Feb 4;19(2):181-92. DOI: 10.1016/j.cmet.2013.12.008. Epub 2014 Jan 16. Longo VD, Mattson MP.

68. Low-Level Mercury in Children: Associations with Sleep Duration and Cytokines TNF-α and IL-6 *Environ Res.* 2014 Oct; 134: 228–232. Published online 2014 Aug 28. DOI: [10.1016/j.envres.2014.07.026] PMCID: PMC4262607 NIHMSID: NIHMS624627 PMID: 25173056. Brooks B. Gump, PhD, MPH, Elena Gabrikova, BS, Kestutis Bendinskas, PhD, Amy K. Dumas, MSEd, Christopher D. Palmer, PhD, Patrick J. Parsons, PhD, and James A. MacKenzie, PhD.

69. Prolonged fasting reduces IGF-1/PKA to promote hematopoietic-stem-cell-based regeneration and reverse immunosuppression. *Cell Stem Cell.* 2014 Jun 5;14(6):810-23. DOI:

10.1016/j.stem.2014.04.014. Cheng CW, Adams GB, Perin L, Wei M, Zhou X, Lam BS, Da Sacco S, Mirisola M, Quinn DI, Dorff TB, Kopchick JJ, Longo VD.

70. Fasting: molecular mechanisms and clinical applications. *Cell Metab.* 2014 Feb 4;19(2):181-92. DOI: 10.1016/j.cmet.2013.12.008. Epub 2014 Jan 16. Longo VD, Mattson MP.

71. Ibid.

72. Ibid.

73. Ibid.

74. Ibid.

75. Prolonged fasting/refeeding promotes hematopoietic stem cell regeneration and rejuvenation. *Rejuvenation Res.* 2014 Aug;17(4):385-9. DOI: 10.1089/rej.2014.1595. Mendelsohn AR, Larrick JW.

76. Episode 108: Water Fasting Done Right. *YouTube Episode 108 for Dr. Dan Pompa* https://drpompa.com/podcasts/108-water-fasting- done-right/ with Dr. Daniel Pompa, Meredith Dykstra, and special guest Dr. Derrick Dempsey.

77. Episode 111: Fasting Tips with Dr. Don Clum. *YouTube Episode 111 for Dr. Dan Pompa* https://drpompa.com/podcasts/111-fasting-tips- dr-don-clum/ With Dr. Daniel Pompa, Meredith Dykstra, and special guest Dr. Don Clum.

78. Fasting: molecular mechanisms and clinical applications. *Cell Metab.* 2014 Feb 4;19(2):181-92. DOI: 10.1016/j.cmet.2013.12.008. Epub 2014 Jan 16. Longo VD, Mattson MP.

79. Autophagy: renovation of cells and tissues. *Cell.* 2011 Nov 11;147(4):728-41. DOI: 10.1016/j.cell.2011.10.026. Mizushima N, Komatsu M.

Chapter 7

1. Prolonged fasting/refeeding promotes hematopoietic stem cell regeneration and rejuvenation. *Rejuvenation Res.* 2014 Aug;17(4):385-9. DOI: 10.1089/rej.2014.1595. Mendelsohn AR, Larrick JW.

2. Beneficial Microbes: The pharmacy in the gut. *Bioengineered.* 2016;7(1):11-20. DOI: 10.1080/21655979.2015.1126015. Linares DM, Ross P, Stanton C.

3. Prolonged fasting/refeeding promotes hematopoietic stem cell regeneration and rejuvenation. *Rejuvenation Res.* 2014 Aug;17(4):385-9. DOI: 10.1089/rej.2014.1595. Mendelsohn AR, Larrick JW.

4. Ibid.

5. Ibid.

6. Role of Low-Level Laser Therapy in Neurorehabilitation. *PM R.* 2010 Dec; 2(12 Suppl 2): S292–S305. DOI: [10.1016/j.pmrj.2010.10.013] PMCID: PMC3065857 NIHMSID: NIHMS281845 PMID: 21172691. Javad T. Hashmi, MD, Ying-Ying Huang, MD, Bushra Z. Osmani, MD, Sulbha K. Sharma, PhD, Margaret A. Naeser, PhD, LAc, and Michael R. Hamblin, PhD.

7. Emerging concepts in bioenergetics and cancer research: metabolic flexibility, coupling, symbiosis, switch, oxidative tumors, metabolic remodeling, signaling and bioenergetic therapy. *Int J Biochem Cell Biol.* 2015 Feb;59:167-81. DOI: 0.1016/j.biocel.2014.12.008. Epub 2014 Dec 24 Obre E1, Rossignol R2.

8. Prolonged fasting reduces IGF-1/PKA to promote hematopoietic-stem-cell-based regeneration and reverse immunosuppression. *Cell Stem Cell.* 2014 Jun 5;14(6):810-23. DOI: 10.1016/j.stem.2014.04.014. Cheng CW, Adams GB, Perin L, Wei M, Zhou X, Lam BS, Da Sacco S, Mirisola M, Quinn DI, Dorff TB, Kopchick JJ, Longo VD.

9. Fasting: molecular mechanisms and clinical applications. *Cell Metab.* 2014 Feb 4;19(2):181-92. DOI: 10.1016/j.cmet.2013.12.008. Epub 2014 Jan 16. Longo VD, Mattson MP.

APPENDIX

MORE ON THE ROLE OF STEM CELLS IN THE HUMAN BODY AND HOW TO MAXIMIZE THEIR ACTIVITY

In the introduction, we established that stem cells are the body's base raw materials it uses to create new tissue and maintain it over time. However, there are several diverse types of stem cells that each serve a slightly different purpose at various stages of a person's life. We categorized the order based on their "potency" or level at which they can repair and form new tissues.

The more primitive cells, like the ones present in the embryonic stage of development, have the greatest ability to repair because they are so youthful and hold the capacity to eventually create a full human body out of an embryo. As a person develops, these cells branch off and create less potent adult stem cells. These are the cells responsible for the lifelong process of cellular healing. There are five main categories of stem cells, and they are:

- **Totipotent**—the ability to differentiate into all possible cell types. Examples are the zygote formed at egg fertilization and the first few cells that result from the division of the zygote.

- **Pluripotent**—the ability to differentiate into almost all cell types. Examples include embryonic stem cells and cells derived from the mesoderm, endoderm, and ectoderm germ layers formed in the beginning stages of embryonic stem cell differentiation.

- **Multipotent**—the ability to differentiate into a closely related family of cells. Examples include mesenchymal and hematopoietic (adult) stem cells that can become red and white blood cells or platelets. They can also signal other cell types to repair themselves.

- **Oligopotent**—the ability to differentiate into a few cells. Examples include (adult) lymphoid or myeloid stem cells.

- **Unipotent**—the ability to only produce cells of their type but have the property of self-renewal required for labeling as a stem cell. Examples include (adult) muscle stem cells.

Although all these types vary in potency, all stem cells have two major paths they can take in their life cycle: Differentiation, which we just discussed, and self-replication.

Self-replication is when the cell makes copies of itself, done in tissue all over the body, to build populations of stem cells for current and later use. Think of it as a bank account that your body draws from for constant maintenance and healing throughout life. Every time stress or injury occurs, the body draws from this bank account, and the available stem cells will release to the damaged areas. They then either secrete signals to stimulate the tissue to repair itself or differentiate and become new cells of that tissue type to replace the lost cells.

When a person undergoes the aging process or consistent long-term stress related to an injury of any kind, their available stem cells must constantly go into "differentiate mode" to keep up with the accumulating damage and perpetual cell loss. Over time, this depletes the person's bank account because more cells are to differentiate than are left behind to self-replicate to keep the bank account full. This stem cell depletion leads to accelerated aging and biological deterioration on every level.

When stem cell populations get too low, the person can almost completely lose the ability to heal and optimize every cell in the body. You are cells. So, if your cells don't work right, you don't work right. The main point is that all cellular healing is a stem cell-mediated process. Maximizing stem cell activity within the body is the key to total health optimization.

So, the next question is, how can we harness the power of stem cells to build cellular resilience, prevent disease, and maximize total performance? This question brings us back to my core philosophy. Remove the interference, then support the innate intelligence with a multi-therapeutic approach. There are many lifestyle changes, dietary shifts, supplements, therapies, and modalities that are all effective. However, we have seen the greatest clinical results with a few strategies, especially when used together. The synergy that comes from integrating it all into a practical system is always where the biggest breakthroughs occur.

FASTING AND FASTING MIMICKING DIETS HOW THEY LEAD TO THE PRODUCTION OF NEW STEM CELLS

To understand how fasting leads to increased stem cell production, you must understand the Recycle/Renewal Principle I introduced you to in this book. Recycling and renewing are the two main steps or phases of the cellular healing and maintenance process. They are two sides of the same coin and are both equally important.

Recycling is the removal of biological interference by breaking down and clearing old damaged cells and impurities. The scientific term for this process is autophagy. This process is the first step of any healing process and must occur to create a hospitable terrain and make room for new healthy cells.

Then comes renewal, which is the creation of new stem cells that differentiate to form new healthy cells to replace the old damaged cells that have just been cleared out and driven by a pathway in the body called mTOR—a pathway that stimulates the growth and recovery of new cells. I like to compare this process to building a new house. If you're looking to build a new house on a property with an old house already present, the first thing you must do is bring in a crew to break down the old house. Then you must clear the debris and create a strong, stable foundation. After that, you assemble the highest quality materials you can find and build the new house.

The body must go through a similar process to renew its tissues and heal. The goal is renewal. To get there, you must effectively go through the recycle phase. Recycling is the path to renewal. The body primarily activates autophagy as an adaptation in times where little to no food is available to use as fuel. Therefore, innate intelligence will selectively recycle bad tissue and stored body fat into usable energy for survival. This both feeds the body and clears out the bad cells to make room for new ones.

Then it is the mTOR pathway that activates all these new cells to grow. Therefore, it is crucial for individuals to maintain a cyclical balance between recycling and renewing by going through times of famine and times of feasting. Fasting and fasting mimicking diets (carbohydrate and protein- restricted diets) are the primary strategies that we use in our protocols to maximize this recycling. Feasting with the right foods at the right time is what helps maximize the renewal of your cells.

However, most people struggle when first implementing carbohydrate- restricted diets and especially fasting because their bodies are mainly burning carbohydrates as a fuel source. It takes time to retrain the body to burn fat as the main fuel source so that the ketogenic diet and even fasting become easy and doable for most people. Since fat-burning and recycling occur together, assistance with becoming fully fat adapted and being able to fast periodically are two of the main objectives of this book.

HERBS AND OTHER SUPPLEMENTS

Western medical systems rarely use herbs, and if they do, they are rarely applied specifically to enhance regeneration. However, Eastern medical systems have been using herbs for regenerative purposes for centuries. Most of the herbs from Chinese and Ayurvedic medicine have today withstood the scrutiny of the modern scientific lens by being shown in countless studies to enhance the body's creation and utilization of stem cells. Because of their amazing effects on stem cell enhancement, they are an extra tool to use in conjunction with the rest of the strategies in this book.

We use many of these tonic herbs either alone or in formulas to maximize stem cell activity and thus the whole healing process. They are a great compliment to standard healthy foods before and after a fast during refeeding. They are the "icing on the cake" when it comes to nutritional strategies and is a great adjunct to a foundation of standard healthy foods.

HOW TONIC HERBS ENHANCE STEM CELL ACTIVITY

As we learned previously, it is the complex action of a vast array of living constituents within tonic herbs that is responsible for their therapeutic action and gives some of them the ability to assist our body in its production of stem cells. We refer to the sum of all these synergistic medicinal constituents as the plant's living matrix.

Think of this plant matrix like a musical orchestra. Each one of its many active constituents is like a single instrument in the arrangement. There are a whole host of different instruments, all with distinct parts to play. Some are much more *active* or play much louder than others. Some play the melody or a more significant role in the overall sound or *activity* of the group. Some instruments are there to support and elevate the more central ones to bring depth and balance to the overall sound. So, in the same way, the plant matrix of medicinal herbs is a composition of many synergistic constituents that together create the overall balanced action or essence of the plant. The same thing goes for the living matrix inside every living organism, such as the regenerative matrix inside the human body that I spoke of in the introduction of this book.

Here are some additional herbs thoroughly researched for their ability to enhance the body's stem cell activity:

- Prepared Rehmannia (Rehmannia glutinosa)

- Prepared He Shou Wu (Polygonum multiflorum)

- Dendrobium Stem Extract (Dendrobium nobile)

- Deer Placenta (Cervus nippon timminck)

- Ligustrum (Ligustrum lucidium)

- White Peony (Paeonia lactiflora)

- Polyrachis Ant Extract (Polyrhachis vicina roger)

- Salvia root (Salvia miltiorrhiza)

- Aged wild American Ginseng (Panax quinquefolius)

- Shilajit (Asphaltum punjabianum)

- Wild Siberian Chaga (Inonotus obliquus)
- Goji Berry Extract (Lycium barbarum)
- Licorice root Extract (Glycyrrhiza glabra)
- Chinese Skullcap (Scutellaria baicalensis)
- Wild Red Reishi Mushroom (Ganoderma lucidum)
- Wild Astragalus Root (Astragalus propinquus)
- Aged Wild Red Panax Ginseng (matured for eight years minimum)
- Wild Cistanche Stem (Cistanche deserticola)
- Deer Antler Velvet (Cervus nippon)
- Wild Tibetan Rhodiola (Rhodiola sacra)
- Horny Goat Weed (Epimedium grandiflorum)
- Eucommia Bark (Eucommia ulmoides)
- Morinda Root (Morinda officinalis)
- Ligusticum Root (Ligusticum chuanxiong)
- Nettle Root (Urtica dioica)
- Cinnamon Bark (Cinnamomum cassia)
- Cordyceps sinenses
- Schisandra Fruit (Schisandra chinensis)
- Cuscuta Seed (Cuscuta chinensis)
- Cornus Fruit (Cornus officinalis)
- Wild Siberian Ginseng Root (Acanthopanax senticosus)
- Polygala Root (Polygala tenuifolia)
- Longan Fruit (Dimocarpus longan)
- Mucuna pruriens

ADDITIONAL SUPPLEMENTS AND SUPERFOODS

These are additional unique nutrient-dense foods and micronutrient supplements that either directly or indirectly support stem cell activity:

- Colostrum (bovine or goat)
- Acai Berry Extract (Euterpe oleracea)
- Wild Harvested Organic Klamath Lake Blue Green Algae (Aphanizomenon flos-aqae)
- Ecuadorian Glacial Water Grown Spirulina
- Green and Red Marine Phytoplankton
- Wild Organic Wakame Flucoidan Extract from Patagonia
- Chlorella (Chlorella vulgaris)
- Noni Fruit (Morinda citrifolia)
- Green Tea Extract (Camellia sinensis)
- Atlantic and Pacific Kelp
- Irish Moss (Chondrus crispus)
- Moringa Leaf Extract (Moringa oleifera)
- Blueberry Extract
- Turmeric (Curcuma longa)
- Vitamin B6 (Pyridoxine HCL)
- Vitamin B12 (Methylcobalamin)
- Folate (5MTHF)
- Magnesium (Malate)
- Iron
- Vitamin C
- Molybdenum (Chelate)

- D-Biotin

- Zinc (Chelate)

- Selenium (Selenomethionine)

- Chromium (4-Hydroxyisoleucinate)

- Manganese (Chelate)

- L- Carnosine

- Vitamin D3

- Copper (Chelate)

- Potassium (Dipotassium phosphate)

- Acetyl-l-Carnitine

- Alpha Lipoic Acid

- Niagen (Nicotinamide riboside)

- COQ10

- Trans-Resveratrol

One main thing to consider when purchasing these supplements is that there is a MASSIVE variation in quality and potency on the market of all these ingredients but especially herbs and superfoods. Growth/harvesting methods, processing methods (drying, extracting), storage methods (preservation), and available forms (for absorbability) are all serious things to consider when sourcing these. Most large commercial supplement manufacturers today have little to no expertise in these areas, which has led to a supplement industry with very few herbs and foods that have the full therapeutic potential for which they are traditionally known. We have recently formulated a product called Cell ReNu that contains all these listed ingredients from what we consider to be the best sources in the world.

RED AND INFRARED LIGHT THERAPY
(PHOTOBIOMODULATION)

Light therapy is a non-invasive method of treatment exposing the selected body area to red or infrared light at varying intensities, which stimulates the cells and tissues and quickens the healing process. Doctors, dentists, physical therapists, and other medical professionals use light therapy in a variety of ways. Over the past decade, lasers and light-based systems have been well- studied and have become a common modality to treat a wide variety of conditions and health problems, including sports injuries, inflammatory conditions, and skin conditions. Current researchers are further expanding the scope of therapeutic use for light therapy as a treatment option for those with neurodegenerative disorders. Also, studies suggest that low-level laser therapy is effective on pain, muscle spasm, morning stiffness, burns, carpal tunnel, and fibromyalgia.

BENEFITS OF LOW-LEVEL LASER THERAPY

Clinical experience shows that low-level laser therapy for several conditions and issues include the following benefits:

- Growth factor response within cells and tissues because of increased ATP and protein synthesis.

- Pain relief because of increased endorphin and serotonin release.

- Increased lymphatic drainage activity and strengthening of immune system response.

- Reduction in inflammation by suppressing inflammatory enzymes that create swelling, redness, pain.

- Aids in tissue repairs like ligament sprains and strains.

- Faster bone repair by stimulating fibroblastic and osteoblastic proliferation.

- Precise stimulation of acupuncture points and energy meridians.

Low-level laser therapy works by stimulating cellular growth and rejuvenation to the applied area. Applied by a special laser beam generator, a low-intensity laser applied to the exposed body produces photon energy.

This energy transforms into biochemical energy, and the cumulative effect after subsequent sessions at set intervals restores the normal functioning of the cells.

Once the light energy passes through the layers of skin and reaches the target area, it is absorbed and interacts with the light-sensitive elements in the cell. This process can is comparable photosynthesis in plants—the absorption of sunlight absorbed, which is then converted to usable energy so the plant can grow. These benefits that ensue are a result of amplified and synchronized infrared light (laser beam) at a certain wavelength (600– 1000 nm) that triggers the cellular and biochemical process, including ATP and collagen production and increased blood flow to the affected area.

In other words, low-level laser therapy works on two basic principles: It increases cellular regeneration and increases cellular communication. When laser light is absorbed by living cells, it triggers biological reactions that stimulate the production of a variety of chemicals within the body that are then released and carried by the blood and lymphatic flow to other parts of the system. It is important to note that the lasers do not induce any temperature change in the body's tissues.

There are five distinct effects associated with low-level laser therapy:

- Growth factor response within cells and tissue because of increased ATP and protein synthesis.

- Improved cell proliferation; change in cell membrane permeability to calcium uptake.

- Pain relief because of increased endorphin and serotonin release plus suppression of nociceptive action.

- Strengthening of immune system response via increasing levels of lymphocyte activity and through a newly researched mechanism.

- Stimulation of acupuncture points.

Treatments can last as little as five minutes, or as much as twenty minutes and most people feel nothing at all during them, although some feel a slight tingling sensation because of the increased blood flow to the treated area. The actual effect of laser therapy begins at the time of treatment, but generally only becomes noticeable several hours or even days after. Patients often must return to the doctor for treatment numerous times to achieve long-term success, depending on the severity and duration of the condition.

PULSED ELECTROMAGNETIC FIELD THERAPY (PEMF)

Pulsed Electromagnetic Field Therapy (PEMF or PEMT) is a non-invasive, painless treatment for various injuries, bone-related conditions and pains, and overall recovery. The treatment works by emitting a pulsating, varying intensity, and frequency electromagnetic field, usually coming from a solenoid placed around the patient. The application of pulsed magnetic fields has, through research findings, been shown to help the body to restore normal potentials at an accelerated rate, thus aiding the healing of most wounds, regenerating tissue, and reducing swelling faster.

Pulsed electromagnetic field therapy replicates the Earth's natural magnetic field, to which we were once strongly connected. Over time, this magnetic field has gotten weaker (an estimated 10% weaker since the 19th century), and because of industrialization and modernization, we are separated further from the Earth's natural magnetic field. The therapy originated from NASA's research involving the benefits of pulsed electromagnetic fields on astronauts for fatigue, depression, bone loss, and other symptoms following even short trips to outer space. Scientists discovered that the cause was because of astronauts being without this beneficial natural field emanating from our Earth.

In 1979 the FDA approved pulsed electromagnetic field therapy specifically for the healing of nonunion fractures, which came after a Columbia University study that was encouraged by NASA and has recently gained attention in the U.S (even appearing as a segment on the Dr. Oz Show). The value of pulsed electromagnetic field therapy has been shown to cover a wide range of conditions, with well-documented trials conducted by hospitals, rheumatologists, physiotherapists, and neurologists.

HERE'S HOW IT WORKS

Pulsed electromagnetic field devices deliver beneficial, health-enhancing fields and frequencies to the cells, addressing the impaired chemistry and stimulating the proper functioning of the cells. As they pass through, they stimulate most of the electrical and chemical processes in the tissues and are specifically designed to positively support cellular energy, resulting in better cellular health and function.

A large benefit of pulsed electromagnetic field therapy is that there are absolutely no side-effects and treatment takes approximately twenty to thirty minutes. Pulsed electromagnetic field therapy improves blood circulation and increases oxygen distribution around the body (when blood cells are stacked together, they are not working to their full potential), making it a useful and non-invasive therapeutic option for pain relief and post-injury healing. PEMF also encourages the blood cells to spread out and reduce plaque in the bloodstream to increase blood viscosity.

HYPERBARIC OXYGEN THERAPY

Hyperbaric oxygen therapy is also great at enhancing stem cell activity in the body. It is used to treat several health conditions, including:

- Severe anemia
- Brain abscess
- Arterial gas embolism (bubbles of air in your blood vessels)
- Burn injuries
- Decompression sickness
- Carbon monoxide poisoning
- Crush injuries
- Sudden deafness
- Gangrene of the tissues
- Infection of skin and bone that causes necrosis (tissue death)
- Skin graft or skin flap at risk for tissue death
- Sudden and painless vision loss

The increased oxygen that builds up in all the bodily fluids during hyperbaric therapy enhances the ability of white blood cells to kill bacteria, reduces swelling and allows new blood vessels to grow more rapidly into the affected areas. It is a simple, non-invasive, and painless treatment.

We have known that healing many areas of the body cannot take place without appropriate oxygen levels in the tissue. Most illnesses and injuries occur and often linger, at the cellular or tissue level. In many cases, such as circulatory problems, non-healing wounds, and strokes. Adequate oxygen cannot reach the damaged area, and the body's natural healing ability is unable to function properly. Hyperbaric oxygen therapy provides this extra oxygen naturally and with minimal side effects. However, HBOT's therapeutic effects aren't just because of the increased oxygen availability that it provides to the cells.

In 2008, there were advances in mass DNA analysis techniques developed that created a revelatory understanding of HBOT in the scientific community. In 2008, Dr. Cassandra Godman and colleagues found that a single hyperbaric treatment to the human cells that line all our blood vessel turns on or turns off over 8,000 genes in the twenty-four hours following the single treatment. If the cells receive another treatment at twenty-four hours, even more, genes are activated, and the cells begin to roll up and form new small blood vessels. Furthermore, they found that the genes that were turned on are those genes which code for growth and repair hormones and the anti-inflammatory genes. The genes turned off were the pro-inflammatory genes and those that code for cell death.

Other research followed and found that various pressures turn on different and overlapping sets of genes and various levels of oxygen turn on different and overlapping sets of genes. Oxygen was responsible mostly for turning on the genes and pressure for turning off the genes.

Essentially, hyperbaric oxygen therapy is the oldest, most enduring, most effective, and most extensive gene therapy known to man. Moreover, it's organic. Each time a patient undergoes a hyperbaric treatment, the physician is playing a symphony with their genes using different pressures and different amounts of oxygen.

So, because of its profound implications, let's look at this again: when oxygen is under pressure, it acts like a drug, and has drug-like effects on the DNA and other components of each cell, bringing about permanent changes in the cell and surrounding tissue. The actual increase in pressure alone is doing the same thing. Over the decades of experimentation with HBOT, we've discovered that it's "secret of success" is its cumulative effect, meaning that after twenty-five to thirty-five treatments, the body's tissues permanently changed.

At the same time, HBOT also has a host of other effects. In particular, and perhaps most important is that a variety of studies have shown that HBOT seems to recruit stem cells to wounded areas. In using HBOT, genes are stimulated to produce growth and repair hormones simultaneously with stem cells acting as a stimulus to tissue regeneration, and this is what makes HBOT such a versatile treatment.

In the treatment of acute conditions, HBOT also affects the patient's DNA. Evidence points to its ability to reverse injury to the DNA or overcome a type of freeze put on the DNA from various insults. It's been my experience that when people understand the treatment in terms of using oxygen as a drug, they quickly open their minds to the idea that the treatment has far-reaching implications.

For many people, the next logical question is, "What conditions can we help by using hyperbaric oxygen therapy?" The short answer is that HBOT is useful for conditions caused or aggravated by reduced oxygen levels in the tissues, and other forms of injury. As you can see, this covers the enormous ground.

Hyperbaric oxygen therapy improves the quality of life of the patient in many areas when standard medicine is not working. Many conditions such as stroke, cerebral palsy, head injuries, and chronic fatigue have responded favorably to HBOT.

STEM CELL THERAPY

We have already learned about stem cell therapy and its profound potential as the foundation of medicine in the future. It is the most powerful strategy on this list because it directly allows you to increase the number of stem cells in your body very quickly. Although this can be an extremely powerful intervention for anyone, there are four main groups of people who will most likely benefit the most by adding stem cell therapy to their health and wellness plan.

The Elderly: As we age, our stem cells also age, leading them to become less and less potent as time goes on. After around the age of forty, our stem cell function starts to decline, and so does our ability to create new stem cells. Even the new stem cells created are slightly less potent than the ones created when we were younger.

By age eighty, our stem cells have lost a significant degree of their original potency, and our ability to produce new stem cells is far less than that of a young person. As we age, we also lose growth factors and other important signaling molecules that activate stem cells and mobilize them into circulation to reach areas that need repair. Anyone over forty can get a significant added benefit by seeking out the stem cell therapies that use younger cells or just put more of their stem cells into circulation and damaged tissues.

Those with Compromised Health: Anyone with a chronic degenerative disease can potentially benefit from receiving injections of extra stem cells, especially those with very significantly progressed degeneration where there is extensive cellular damage that has built up over many years. In these cases, the individual's stem cells are usually also compromised or damaged from being subjected to all the same environmental factors that are driving the disease process.

Previously I mentioned that self-replication and differentiation are the two main paths that stem cells can take in their life cycle. When a person undergoes the aging process or consistent long-term stress-related injury of any kind (like an injury that occurs in degenerative disease), their available stem cells must go into "differentiate mode" to keep up with the accumulating damage and perpetual cell loss. Over time this depletes the person's stem cell reservoir as more cells go to differentiate than are left behind to self-replicate and replenish the reserve. For these individuals, stem cell therapy can help them gain leverage over the disease process by making up for the deficit in healthy viable stem cells and supply the extra stem cells and signaling factors that may be necessary to repair the extensive damage in the body's tissues.

Those with Acute Injuries: Stem cells are being used in clinics around the world to help patients recover from many acute injuries. Individuals with everything from joint injuries to head trauma can benefit greatly from the large numbers of stem cells given intravenously or injected directly into the injury site.

Those Seeking Anti-Aging Effects and Total Health Optimization: Even if a person isn't in the middle of a serious disease process, they still might be able to receive benefit from stem cell therapy. Many health- conscious individuals around the world are seeking out these treatments for extra regenerative support to try to bring their health to the next level, slow and potentially reverse the aging process. Many who are doing this are reporting a vast array of positive results such as increased mental clarity, faster recovery, better sleep, increased energy, and better overall vitality.

ADDITIONAL INFORMATION

Core Cellular Package: http://corecellular.stemnomicguide.com

Proper cell function is a prerequisite to the body being able to heal itself, so nutrients must be able to dock with cell membrane receptors, enter the cell, and be useable toward cellular metabolic processes so that the cellular proteins can guide the cells activities and epigenetic expressions and avoid the expression of disease. This program addresses key factors of cellular activities including membrane fluidity, antioxidant usage, inflammation, methylation, ATP energy, repair of chromosomes and telomeres, and detoxification.

KetoSports MCT Oil: http://mctoil.stemnomicguide.com

MCT oil is a well-known keto and low-carb aid that increases blood ketone levels and is useable in a variety of applications, including supplementation and cooking. Most commercially available MCT oils are a combination of C8 and C10 in a 60:40 ratio and derived from sources such as coconut or palm oil. Both C8 and C10 provide increased ketone levels; however, C8 has proven to be the superior choice. C8 has been shown to increase blood ketone levels by a greater amount than its counterpart, by almost twofold, and C8 is ten times less likely to store as body fat by the liver. So, we bottled this powerful aid into 12-ounce bottles. This product is clear and tasteless.

KetoSports Keto Force: http://ketoforce.stemnomicguide.com

Keto Force contains the exogenous ketone body beta-hydroxybutyrate (BHB) in sodium and potassium salt form. Ingestion of Keto Force will raise the levels of blood ketones (BHB and AcAc) for 2.5-3.0 hours after ingestion. When taken within fifteen minutes before exercise, this product has been shown to decrease the amount of oxygen consumed at a given power output.

benaGene™: http://benagene.stemnomicguide.com

benaGene™ contains patented "Thermally Stabilized Oxaloacetate" and Vitamin. While you may be familiar with Vitamin C, oxaloacetate is a natural energy molecule critical to human metabolism and proper cellular function. benaGene supplies your body with additional oxaloacetate.

Fasting Trio: http://fastingtrio.stemnomicguide.com

The three products found in this package support during a period of fasting. Fasting offers amazing benefits for repair and improved health, and we want you to be comfortable during your journey to optimize your results.

Fastonic: http://fastonic.stemnomicguide.com

Fastonic is one of our fasting favorites. This product provides H2 to the body. This molecule provides the body with tons of benefits. Fastonic can promote a healthy balance of oxidative stress, neutralizing only the most harmful free radical into water. It supports glucose homeostasis, decreases appetite, and stabilizes cholesterol. It helps to promote healthy functioning of the inflammation system. Fastonic also supports cognitive function allowing for increased mental clarity, while reducing fatigue associated with fasting.

Colostrum: http://colostrum.stemnomicguide.com

Colostrum, often called "Immune-Milk," is one of the most diverse whole- food supplements available today. Packed with protein and containing all essential fats, Surthrival Colostrum boasts an impressive nutrient suite of vitamins, minerals, probiotics, growth factors, and amino acids. Versatile, simple to use, and rich-and-creamy tasting, Colostrum is the perfect solution and support system to achieve your health objectives. So, whether you're working your movement game hard, or trying to establish a healthy baseline; Colostrum is your "Plan A" for an upgraded life.

www.drpompa.com

Our philosophy is simple. Healing can come only from inside-out, never from outside-in, and the true doctor of the future must be a doctor who removes the interferences and lets the body do the healing.

ABOUT THE AUTHOR AND HIS WORK

Dr. Daniel Pompa, PSc.D., is a global health leader and innovator on a mission to educate practitioners and the public on the origins of inflammation-driven diseases, cellular detoxification, fasting strategies, and diet variation principles. Although trained as a chiropractor, his authority comes from the victory within his battle, having overcome a neurotoxic illness rooted in heavy metal poisoning.

Dr. Pompa is known for using and developing unique cellular detoxification strategies. For the past two decades, he has been relentlessly studying, practicing, and teaching True Cellular Detox™ to many around the world. He also hosts a podcast called *Cellular Healing TV*, and an internet radio show known as *Health Hunters Radio.*

Dr. Pompa and his wife, Merily, have their own story to tell as they have raised five children—three of their own and two they adopted after a tragedy in Merily's family. After a story that only God could write, they embraced and endured significant challenges. Through their faith, they embarked on a journey that not only included relocating from Pittsburgh, PA, to Park City, UT, but also a new chapter of life for the whole Pompa family. The blog,

From Pain to Purpose isn't just a way of attaching purpose to Dr. Pompa's sickness and their family's battle, but it is a statement of faith that has gained traction around the world as they openly share that hope and faith with all who know them.

Research interests include a therapeutic application of the ketogenic diet, fasting, ancestral-based health approaches, and cellular healing and detoxification.

Dr. Pompa coaches health practitioners on innovative solutions to fixing cellular dysfunction and currently has a wait-list of private clients. Past presentations range from *Ancient Healing Secrets*, and *The Ins and Outs of Ketosis: Clinical Wisdom*, to his personal story, *From Pain to Purpose to Promise.*

Author of *The Cellular Healing Diet.*

NOTABLE INTERVIEWS AND PODCASTS

Robert Scott Bell; Zach Bush, MD; Dominic D'Agostino, MD; Billy DeMoss, MD; Jason Fung, MD; Patrick Gentempo, MD; Ben Greenfield, MD; David Kennedy;

Jack Kruse, MD; Bruce Lipton, MD; Joe Mercola, MD; Jordan Rubin; Barry Sears, MD; Stephanie Seneff, MD; Thomas Seyfried, Ph.D.; Jeff Volek, MD; Terry Wahls, MD; Naomi Whittle; Jack Wolfson, MD.

LIVE PRESENTATIONS

Dr. Pompa's Story: *From Pain to Purpose* (Public Audience)

Bulletproof Presentation (Public Audience)

Cal Jam Conference Stage Video (Health Practitioner Audience)

Mitochondrial Epidemic (Health Practitioner Audience)

Diet Variation (Health Practitioner Audience)

Fasting (Health Practitioner Audience)

EDUCATION

Life University, Atlanta, GA—Doctor of Chiropractic, 1995; Summa Cum Laude, Class Salutatorian

University of Pittsburgh, Pittsburgh, PA—Bachelor of Science, 1989; Honors, Class Salutatorian

SOCIAL MEDIA

https://cellularhealing.tv/welcome-to-chtv

Every Friday at 10 am (EST), Dr. Dan Pompa, Warren Phillips, and guest health experts discuss cellular healing solutions and strategies that will transform your life and how you view health. Healing and death begin on the cell membrane, so that means when you learn how to heal the cell, you will get well.

https://hcfseminars.com

Health Centers of the Future (HFC) Seminars birthed out of a desire to educate and train health care practitioners, chiropractors, students, and medical doctors who will stand in the gap between the modern day epidemic of disease and the patients they serve, enabling them to offer true answers to the question, "Why am I sick?"

HCF Seminars does not require massive marketing efforts of the practitioner to get new patients. It does, however, require one thing: To see your clients get completely well.

HCF Seminars teaches their protocols and marketing strategies to hundreds of doctors around the world in cities such as Atlanta, Las Vegas, New York, and Minneapolis year-round. These seminars feature a multitude of speakers including Daniel Pompa, D.PSc; Warren Phillips; David Asarnow; and health experts such as Alan R Vinitsky, MD; Martin L Pall Ph.D.; Patrick Gentempo, DC; Dr. Shayne Morris, Ph.D. and many more.

https://revelationhealth.com

Dr. Pompa's favorite supplement shop! Revelation Health provides therapeutic grade supplements, organic foods, healthy home products, and natural body care, using only the safest ingredients, approved, and utilized by our network of physicians across the country. These exclusive product lines include Systemic Formulas, 180° Solutions™, Designs for Health®, NuMedica, Complimentary Prescriptions (SFI), SFI, Prescript-Assist, Interplexus, Byron White, BodyBio, NutraMedix, CytoDetox®, Natural Radiance, Simple Life Mom, Remedy Link, Stevita, Virgin Pacific Water, AllerAir, World Nutrition, and many more.

Most of these select lines require a qualified physician on staff to implement correct usage and to dose to ensure the greatest outcomes. Along with practitioners on staff, we have health coaches certified by the American Association of Drugless Practitioners (AADP). They are available to answer your questions about health and offer weight loss and detoxification strategies and solutions to help you feel and look your best. We're pleased to provide our customers with only the highest quality products to confront the maze of new millennium diseases threatening the health of our nation. We specialize in creating natural support strategies for weight loss, diabetes, thyroid disorders, low energy, chronic pain, and digestive challenges.

ADVANCE PRAISE FOR *BEYOND FASTING*

"Dr. Pompa has been a pioneer in the use of diet and fasting in improving health and wellness. He shares his valuable experience in this must-read book."

- DR. JASON FUNG, author of *The Complete Guide to Fasting*

"When we filmed Dan about fasting, ketosis, and the direct effects on stem cell regeneration for our pain and stem cell documentary, I told him that I thought this really should be his next book. The research is so clear on what a powerful effect this has, but the gap between research and clinical is often 20 years or more, meaning your doctor won't know the information the research is showing today for 20 years! Dan's Stemnomic diet bridges that 20-year gap and makes this incredible new research available today in an easy- to- follow program for the millions of people who so desperately need it."

- JEFF HAYES, filmmaker and director of *The Real Skinny on Fat*

"Research tells us that stress, age, poor diet, and environmental toxins are some of the main culprits that are driving these conditions. All these issues cause inflammation and deplete us of our precious stem cells. Our stem cells are the body's main tools for maintaining youth and the ability to heal from injury or disease. Dr. Pompa provides practical steps each week to prepare you for the fast, plus many adjunctive strategies that increase stem cell activity, stem cell mobilization, and much more."

- BEN GREENFIELD, fitness coach, speaker and author of the New York Times bestseller *Beyond Training: Mastering Endurance, Health and Life*

Dr. Daniel Pompa is a global health leader and innovator on a mission to educate practitioners and the public on the origins of inflammation-driven diseases, cellular detoxification, fasting strategies, and diet variation principles. Although trained as a chiropractor, his authority comes from the victory within his battle, having overcome a neurotoxic illness that was rooted in heavy metal poisoning.